THE REALITY
OF
BREASTFEEDING

by
CATHERINE HOLLAND

Printed by CreateSpace July 2016

A copy of this book is lodged with the Legal Deposit Office at the British Library.

First published by Lifeworks February 1999

ISBN 978-0-9521696-1-1

Cover drawing by Catherine Holland of Anna, at 1 week old.

Dedication

To all those breastfeeding couples who have telephoned me for support, especially those who rang while I was typing, you spurred me on.

And to my three children, now almost all grown up, who were once my bonny breastfed babies.

THE REALITY OF BREASTFEEDING

This is not quite a 'How To' book – more a 'This is Possibly What it Might Feel Like' book – try it and see.

Preface

I have set out in this book to describe the way that breastfeeding works, what you can expect, what the normal variations are, an ideal scenario and some ways to fit nursing into a modern lifestyle. I have drawn on my own breastfeeding experience, that of my friends and those women I have spoken to in the course of counselling calls and visits. I have covered some of the issues that are often missed in the course of preparation for parenthood, mostly because they are things that we might learn from watching other family members raise their children. We think that these things are instinctive but they are not, we miss the opportunity to learn them because we tend to have smaller families, live far away from our extended families and because public breastfeeding is rare here in Britain.

I particularly wish to concentrate on the feelings of parents, their emotional experience: the least prepared area of all.

I apologise for a certain amount of repetition in different sections. The influence of one aspect on another in breastfeeding means that I may have to mention it more than once. I also intend this book to be used as a quick reference for ideas so I want each section to stand alone.

INTRODUCTION

Is Breastfeeding instinctive?
Everybody knows it's natural to breastfeed. So why aren't all the women who want to doing it?
Men think their women will automatically know what to do, the women think they ought to as well. They are horrified if they realize that they don't. Those that do know may not realize that they have copied their skills from women that they have watched. They may not remember the experience if it was long ago, but it stays. Babies instinctively suckle but they expect their mums to know how to hold them and to put them in the correct position to latch on properly. This is a skill

learned from watching others, and if you have never had this opportunity then you simply may not know.

When I was three years old my brother was born. I am the third of four children, all breastfed. I don't remember watching my mother but she tells me I was there at her elbow watching every feed. When I had my own baby I felt my body knew how to hold her and I knew it would work. One of the problems I come across when offering support with breastfeeding is that people do not believe that it works. They do not trust their bodies to work properly. Think about it. Your body knows how to make blood, and just as you can trust your liver or kidneys to work properly today, you can trust your body to nurture your growing baby during pregnancy and to produce the right milk once it is born.

It is a strange fact but it's true that just occasionally I have a phone call from a woman who just needs to know that I have nursed a baby – to show that it is possible.

I guess that Nature expects us to see perhaps forty babies breastfed before we have our own, so that we have a fair amount of experience to draw on of the natural variation of feeding behaviour. An expectation that the system works makes a big difference to women's experience. The belief and wishes of their partners and other members of the family has a great influence. The availability of formula milk also plays a big part. I understand that failure of lactation in other mammals is unknown and as a body function it is more successful than pregnancy. In places where breastfeeding is expected, it works – even where there may be restrictions – on not feeding for the first 24 hours for example.

All new experiences tire us and new parenthood is no exception. The problem that I often encounter is that parents are given completely unrealistic expectations, for example, thinking that a new baby will automatically sleep all night alone. Alternatively they have unrealistic expectations of themselves; that they should be able to be awake and alert six times in the night and all day if the baby needs to be fed. The notion that people sleep with their babies all over the world, let alone here in Britain, seems to be a well kept secret. Babies need their parents in the night and we need to acknowledge this and cater for it if we want our children breastfed and their parents not suffering from guilt and exhaustion.

My point of view

I am sharing what I have learned because I hope that it may help you to relax and enjoy your baby. Remember though that all babies differ, all breastfeeding couples vary. I hope that you will understand from the examples I give that you are the only experts on your baby: that you have to trust yourselves and your bodies to know what is right. Human mothers have been making the ideal milk for their babies for at least 10,000 years. It helps to get this in perspective and to realize that our doubts are more likely to cause a problem than the quality of our milk.

My experience of the way breastfeeding worked for me will suit some mothers and not others. Read what I say as an opinion and then make up your own mind about what feels right for you. I learned as I went along, sometimes the hard way, and I would be pleased to know that someone may benefit from my experience.

Some of the things I learned about that saved a lot of time and trouble were:

Feeding without reference to clocks at all
The baby knowing when it wants to change sides or finish a feed itself
What's right for one baby won't suit another
Avoiding foods myself that caused colic in my fully breastfed baby (in my case cow's milk protein)
Increases in frequency of feeding are temporary
Carrying my baby – around the house, on my bike, everywhere
Breastfeeding in public – discreetly with a shawl
Sleeping with my baby – what all mammals do
Feeding my baby in my sleep
Weaning straight onto adult foods – without puréeing
Night-time nursing in darkness meant no changing of nappies in the night
Babies do not need to cry
A baby never needs to have a bottle
Breastfeeding continues all the time the baby learns to eat other things
Illness brings a temporary return to full scale nursing
Normal variation in feeding pattern is huge

Breastfeeding in the bath is soothing and helps feeding problems

Bottle feeding is never a solution to a breastfeeding problem

I have also learned from the many women by whom I have been telephoned over the years and I pass on all that I have learned so that you may find solutions that work for you.   Some of them are contradictory. Apparently opposite solutions can work with different babies because they are individuals.

Ideal Scenario

Ideally a baby should have access to the breast to feed at anytime and therefore be constantly with its mother. However there is a flexibility in the system which many mothers use if they leave their babies. Alternatively it is possible to take a young baby into all sorts of social and work situations if you plan ahead and ask. I say this because many people assume that breastfeeding stops if a woman returns to work. (see Returning to work and Breastfeeding p.150)

I am aware that some parents are not in a position to be with their children full-time.

This applies to dads more than mums in a way because society accepts that children need their mothers and makes some provision for this. Babies need their dads too and the traditional fathering rôle expects little of men who go out to work for long hours. If men want more involvement they have to actively step out of this stereotypical position. Discussing this with your partner will enable you to learn what each of you would like and what you would like each other to do. This is relevant to breastfeeding because sometimes breastfeeding precipitates a feeling of envy that would not exist if the dad were free to spend more time with his baby.

I shall discuss alternatives for how your baby should be fed while you are not there.

What actually happens (adaptations to situations less than ideal)

Even if you cannot create what you feel are the ideal circumstances for breastfeeding, work out what you can do. Any breastfeeding is better than none. Breastmilk is far better than formula even if your baby cannot have it directly from the breast. Some breastmilk is better than none - if your baby is being mostly formula fed and you wonder if it is worth struggling with mixed feeding but wish your baby still to be partially breastfed.

It is possible to express milk if you cannot feed your baby straightaway once born.

It is possible to return to breastfeeding when a baby has been formula fed. This is easiest while the baby is under four weeks old. If you want to breastfeed, you can. It is even possible to breastfeed an adopted baby (see under Special Circumstances : Adoption p.154). For more information about these circumstances consult Breastfeeding Counsellors – details under Breastfeeding Organisations. The La Leche League have a resource book covering special circumstances – try the library or their address.

HOW BREASTFEEDING WORKS

Generally speaking rules are antithesis to breastfeeding. I think probably "Trust Your Baby" would be my suggestion. However there are some things you need to know about how the system works. I describe them below in more detail.

Three things you need to know:

1. The demand creates the supply.
2. Correct latching on to the breast is important.
3. Finish the first breast first.

Supply and Demand

The amount of milk a breastfeeding mother produces is dictated by the sucking of the baby, or babies, she is nursing. Whatever the baby takes is replaced. The feedback mechanism is direct and the response fairly immediate. It relies upon the baby having access to the breast when it asks either by sucking its fist or opening its mouth hopefully and turning towards the mother (rooting reflex). The baby needs to be able to spend as much time as it wants to at the breast as often as it wants to. The normal variation for this is enormous. There is a certain amount of flexibility in the timing; you don't have to get it right every time. But the practice of regulating feeds over the last thirty years has caused many women in Britain to believe that they cannot breastfeed. For example it has been discovered by research that the minimum number of breastfeeds a day to maintain a supply is five. For many years women were told to feed four hourly. This means that they were only just above that minimum level, and many found their supply dwindled. They were then advised to supplement with formula which reduced the baby's appetite at the breast and lowered the supply of breastmilk further. The solution when there is not enough milk is to nurse the baby more often until the supply increases to satisfy the baby. Many people find it hard to believe that when a breastfed baby has had enough to eat it will come off the breast of its own ac-cord – usually with a wonderful look of blissful satiation on its face.

The use of dummies or anything else other than the breast to suck on can affect the supply of breast milk. Therefore if you wish to fully breastfeed, you are advised not to use them. Since the word dummy means pretend, and a baby's dummy is a substitute for the breast, you will see that it makes sense for a breastfed baby not to need one. However some breastfeeding mothers do use them once their milk supply is well es-tablished (ie after several months), or if they wish to wean before their baby has outgrown his need to suck. The problem is that you do not know beforehand what

the effect of using a dummy will be on your supply -
and some babies will refuse the breast after being
offered only one bottle.   A recent article in a
breastfeeding newsletter describes how a fully
breastfeeding infant, gaining weight well, became
reluctant to breastfeed after being given a dummy. The
mother was disturbed to find that her baby preferred the
dummy, stopped gaining weight as well and changed
her feeding technique, so the mother now gets sore.
She has worked hard to reestablish her supply several
weeks later.   She wrote the article to warn other
mothers.

It is common for young babies to want to nurse
somewhere between one and three hourly, and not with
the same gap each time.   Unless the breasts are
stimulated they will not continue to produce milk. This
is why women without children do not have milk and
why a mother can relactate if her recently weaned child
becomes ill and returns to nursing.

It takes at least three weeks to get used to being a
parent, to learn your baby's communication signals and
to establish what your baby's feeding habits are. All
this whether you are breastfeeding or not.

Breastfeeding also takes about this length of time to establish and many worried new parents find the extra responsibility of breastfeeding more than they can handle on top of everything else. First I would say that it is best not to make any major life decision during the first few weeks with your new baby. I believe that breastfeeding is one of those decisions that you live with for the rest of your life. I say this because as a breastfeeding counsellor I speak to many grandmothers of grown children, often of the mothers I am counselling at the time, and it is something they always remember – and often regret if they didn't persevere (in getting the help they needed – many tried as well as they could, but received incorrect information). This is an important time in the rôle of supportive 'breastfeeding' fathers. If you know your partner planned to breastfeed before your baby was born and you are having difficulties, resist the temptation to dive for the most expedient solution to getting the baby fed today (a bottle of formula?), and find help. You do not have to struggle on alone. She may be cross with you months later if you don't. This can be an emotional roller coaster of a time for you both and it is the dad's job to stand between the mother and the outside world at this time, to support her in what you know she will be happy with in years to come. Traditionally childbirth is a time when families rally around and support the new parents. Often couples live a long way away from their families. Sometimes their families have only unsuccessful experiences of breastfeeding and feel that it is pointless to try.

Latching on

Some babies take to the breast first time. Others don't. If you have been using nipple shields (which are often advised for nipple soreness and engorgement when correct positioning might be useful, but takes longer), your baby has had bottles or simply does not know how to feed instinctively straight away, you may find yourself with the task of teaching your baby to latch on properly. This seems to be a rather rare expertise and not necessarily known by those who might be expected to have the knowledge. Many mothers who have contacted me have been told by midwives that their babies are latched on properly only to find that the pain they have been experiencing continues. If it hurts there is something wrong.

Suckling involves two actions on the part of the baby:
1. Suction with lips and tongue to hold the nipple and areola in its mouth in the correct position and
2. Milking the breast with the tongue and lower jaw to obtain the milk from the ducts where it is stored.

The breast has to be well into the baby's mouth for the jaw to work and draw out the milk. If the nipple only is taken – which the mother may expect if she has only seen bottle feeding – it will hurt and the baby will not be satisfied. The breast has to be stimulated correctly for the milk to flow, otherwise it would come out when you didn't want it to...

To begin with the baby needs to be held horizontally, body in line with the head thereby supporting the back of the neck, facing and close to the mother's body, usually resting along the forearm. The back of the head must not be touched and left free to move so the baby knows it can breathe. Some mothers are told to push the baby onto the breast. This can end up with a distraught baby who wants to feed but is afraid that he won't be able to breathe.

He needs to be held very close with the nipple pointing to the roof of his mouth, apparently pointing up his nose. Then he can take in the breast with a tip tilt head motion which is characteristic of latching onto the breast with a greater part of the lower breast being taken into the baby's mouth. As he opens his mouth, pull him swiftly slightly (about an inch) towards you so he gets the breast fully into his mouth. Sometimes mothers are taught to hold the breast in a 'scissor' hold (first and second finger each side of the areola) to enable the baby to take the breast when it is tiny, or to support the breast or to enable the baby to breathe. Occasionally it is useful to assist the baby to latch on by lifting the breast up slightly from underneath. Consistent manipulation of the breast can cause blocked ducts and is unnecessary. The baby's nose is designed so that he can breathe even with his face apparently buried in the breast as he feeds – little air gaps exist around the sides of his snub nose – and as long as he is able to freely move his head back, he will pull away to breathe when he needs to. Some mothers are quite upset when they tell me how they have been manhandled by midwives anxious to get the baby latched on. The trick is to wait and keep offering, making sure that he can reach, he will latch on in his own good time.

The changes in position that I suggest most frequently are:

(i) Moving the baby across the mother's body (from elbow towards centre) while in the crook of her arm and

(ii) Pulling the baby closer tucking his body right in close to hers.

For all of this to work and the baby to have a lengthy and satisfying feed can take some time – time that midwives are often not allocated and why I feel that breastfeeding counsellors would be a useful resource within the maternity services.

Many nipples appear flat and if the breast is full the newborn may have difficulty latching on. New babies have such tiny mouths. A glass of iced water held onto the skin at the side of the breast can sometimes cause the skin to feel harder with the cold and enable the baby to latch on. You have to be quick while the effect lasts. Expressing a small amount of milk to soften the breast can also help. Once the breasts have softened after the initial rush of milk and extra blood supply there is usually not so much difficulty in latching on. Babies grow so quickly that the size of their mouth changes and they find the breast easier to grasp. It takes practice.

Mothers feel pressurized to get it right quickly or give formula. The determined ones try again once they get home and often this is the time that I come into contact with them. Many more would be breastfeeding if this help were available sooner.

Mothers I speak to say that they just wish someone had said: "It might take an hour and a half" like I did and at least they would know what they had to do. I believe it takes a young baby about 100 times to learn something new, so each attempt brings you closer to getting your baby latched on. He also gets tired during the process so it quite usual for the baby to have little cat naps during the time you are getting him to latch on properly. Falling asleep at the breast is often seen as a problem, but it is normal, and the baby will either keep nursing gently in its sleep – which is fine – or wake and try again shortly. All the time spent at the breast stimulates supply and every suck by the baby produces milk; towards the end of the feed this is the richest milk producing the most growth and orders the milk supply increase for tomorrow. Remember the only way that the breast knows that more milk needs to be made is by the baby asking for more than it had today.

When you are being supported during this period, make sure common sense prevails. Your baby is not going to starve in the time it takes to learn to feed from the breast and cries of "But he's hungry " do not help you to successfully learn to breastfeed and suggest that breastmilk is not as satisfying for your baby as formula, which is not true.

Finish the first breast first

The milk a baby takes from the breast varies throughout a feed. The milk he gets when he first latches on is called foremilk, it is available straightaway and makes up about a third of the milk available at that time. It is thirst quenching because it is not as fat rich as the hindmilk, which lets down as the baby continues to feed. It is rich in protective substances, particularly antibodies. The baby can stay at the first breast until he has had all the foremilk and then as much of the hindmilk as he needs at that time. Changing from one breast to the other needs to be led by the baby so that he gets the balance of nutrients that he needs. You will know when he wants the other one if he comes off one side and looks around hopefully for food still. If you put him back on the same breast he will probably shout at you.

Many babies fed this way will only want one breast per feed, especially when small. Don't be surprised though if he wants to change this later. He can vary his feeding pattern, if there is a heatwave for example, to switching to the other breast quite soon because he is mostly thirsty. The breasts will make more foremilk if the weather is very hot and the baby needs to drink more. This explains why breastfed babies do not need to be given anything other than breast milk; indeed doing so can cause the system to be less effective. It is also much safer to give a baby breast milk in hot climates. I sometimes get a batch of calls during a spell of hot weather, when previously predictable and satisfied babies become frequent nursers. The mothers worry that something is terribly wrong until I point out that we all get thirstier in the summer and they are doing fine.

Let down

The let down is the expression given to the moment after the message from the baby latching onto the breast has been relayed to the brain, the hormone has been released, and the breast reacts by expressing the milk forcefully from the milk sacs through the ducts and out into the baby's mouth. This sensation is usually felt by the mother. Usually it is a tingling sensation. Sometimes it is a burning feeling, and it can be painfully strong. Throughout the duration of breastfeeding the feeling usually lessens, and some women never feel it. It can be an indicator of whether the baby is getting enough to eat. If the baby is unhappy, constantly feeding and dissatisfied and the mother does not feel any letting down, the baby may not be getting enough hind milk to feel full and grow well.

When the baby first takes the breast, he munches a few times to tell the mother's breast that he wants to receive her milk. Then he waits, taking the foremilk that is already present in the ducts. The breast then begins to squirt hindmilk into the baby's mouth after a little while. The normal time interval varies from half a minute to several minutes. It also varies between women, in the same woman at different times and with different babies, if the mother is relaxed, happy with breastfeeding, cold, tense or frightened. I have recently noticed that it is affected by the mothers' relatives anxiety about the baby getting enough milk to thrive … a self-fulfilling prophecy.

Failure to let down adequately is temporary. Sometimes women worry that their milk has dried up, when it appears not to let down. This is a biological response to stress as the frightened mother will stop lactating and move to a safer spot to nurse her young. All over the world women are breastfeeding while they labour or in troubled circumstances, perhaps as refugees. The last thing on their mind is whether they will be able to produce milk. Since they always have, they take it for granted. There was a report in a breastfeeding newsletter by a western mother who was sheltering in an air raid shelter during troubles in Israel. She was nursing her baby while wondering whether a bomb would drop on them all... It put everything into perspective for me, reading her account and realizing what conditions a woman must be able to survive, and keep breastfeeding through.

The effect of breastfeeding also calms a mother and enables her to be protective of her children under threatening circumstances.

During a feed there may be several intervals where the baby sucks, waits, drinks, and sucks and waits again. This is the way that the breast reacts to and produces what the baby needs in each feed. People have a tendency to worry about the fact that the baby does not feed at the same rate throughout a feed and that sometimes it stops and looks around (perhaps while waiting for the let down). Babies do not have the same urgency or fears that they will be underfed if they don't take their milk in a certain time. There is all the time in the world and that is the way it is supposed to work. Again the comparison with bottle feeding is unfortunate. The person holding the bottle is in control, not the baby. While the bottle is tipped up the baby has to swallow or choke. If the person with the bottle is responsive to the baby, they will find that the baby likes to stop for little breaks in its feed too. When a calf feeds from its mother the same process of asking and waiting exists. The young being responsible for the type and amount of milk they take.

Differences between milks

People worry about how much milk their baby is getting. This is to be expected in a society that constantly measures things, and formula does need to be carefully measured: it is dangerous not to. We do not need to know how much breastmilk our babies are getting. The amount and constitution of each feed is dictated by the baby's appetite. It is sad that women do not trust their bodies to produce the right milk; but I suppose it is not surprising given that many civilized women do not trust their own appetite. Human milk is 'weaker' in comparison with cow's milk; it has less fat, it has different protein, it has less salt. But our bodies do this on purpose! Human babies used to die when they were given unmodified cow's milk. Calves grow much faster, and they have smaller brains. All mammals' milks vary, from the tiny shrew to the blue whale, whose milk contains 48% fat – the same as double cream – and whose baby must put on half a ton a week to stay alive in the cold arctic waters. Cow's milk is also not the closest mammal milk to human milk, which I understand is donkey's milk, but cow's milk is available in large quantities and that seems to be why it has been used. Human milk has different proteins, one of which is not present in cow's milk at all, it has different types of fat that are digestible by the human infant and it has a host of protective mechanisms specifically targeted at the needs of the human baby. It is interesting to note that if calves were given human milk they would not survive.

Human babies are designed to grow comparatively slowly; faster weight gain does not, in itself, mean healthier children.

Weight gain

Consistent weight gain is one indication of a healthy infant. There are others such as alertness, contentment, rounded cheeks. The issue of weight gain is sometimes overemphasized above the other signs, and parents are often worried unnecessarily about it.

A consistent weight gain of anything between one ounce and one pound a week can be fine in a fully breastfed baby. It can be useful to discover the parents' weight gain as infants if there is concern. Adults who gained weight slowly as infants are more likely to produce children who follow a similar pattern. Having said this, each baby is different, and within the same family there can be considerable variation. Some breastfed babies gain weight very quickly to begin with and then gain no weight for months on end but grow taller. Some gain more slowly but carry on growing at that rate for years. Logically if a child continued to gain at the rate of growth expected in the first few months of life they would be outrageously large. My brother worked out that if my daughter continued to gain at fourteen ounces a week, she would weigh a ton by the time she was seven years old... My friends' babies gained one ounce a week and continued to do so. My son gained a pound a week at first, weighing thirty pounds at a year, but between eighteen months and three years gained no weight and grew four inches taller. The point I am making is that we can trust the child's appetite and their body to make them grow up into adults in the most suitable way for them. Incidentally, I was told that my daughter was gaining too much weight on my milk. Fortunately I carried on nursing her, having asked what the health visitor proposed I do about it. The problem we have is that breast milk and formula are seen as the same thing and they are not. Plump breastfed babies are designed to withstand infections, during which they may lose up to half their body weight, and survive without permanent damage. The weight that my children put on as chubby infants was converted into growth, and that rounded baby has grown into a tall, slim adult. I would like to suggest that this process of the child being in control of its food contributes to a healthier attitude to eating later; this is certainly true of my children. It is strange in a culture obsessed with weight loss in adults to be so obsessed with weight gain in infants. Maybe there is a connection? It is possible to force a baby to take more from a bottle – first you can push it into their mouth, then the baby has to swallow or it chokes – but you cannot force him to take the breast: it is voluntary action. So worrying about over fat breastfed babies is also inappropriate, as their food intake is self directed and their fat is convertible into growth.

The growth charts used for many years have been based on formula-fed babies. Growth is also not necessarily consistent. Babies tend to have growth spurts and we warn breastfeeding mothers to expect them. When your baby seems much hungrier just when you thought you had got the pattern of feeding he liked sorted out, he is changing it because he needs to grow and has increased his appetite. This means that for a few days he will feed far more often and then settle back into a pattern again, though probably not the same one.

(For information about temporary lack of weight gain see under Illness in the mother p.89)

Differences between breastmilk and formula

If you feel instinctively that formula cannot be as good for your baby as your breastmilk, you are right. I am going to explain some of the reasons why so that you know that your instincts are correct and not just a funny feeling.

I am not going to list all of the known contents of milks but to give an outline.

If you take a look at the side of a can of formula you will see a list of ingredients: the substances and chemicals used to create an artificial attempt at replicating human milk. Some of the ingredients are of animal origin: the base is cow's milk protein for example. Many of the ingredients; such as the oils and sugars, have vegetable origins. Other substances in smaller quantities have been added when deficiencies have become obvious. We have not yet identified all of the constituents of breastmilk. We do not know how many there are to discover, how important they are and we may never know. For example Vitamin D was believed to be absent from human milk because it was not discovered by those looking for it in the fat content as it is in cow's milk. Breastfed babies were for a while considered to be in danger of deficiency until a different type was discovered in the whey portion because it was water soluble. This is a good example of how cow's milk is considered as the yardstick by which to measure human milk when it is completely inappropriate; any more than it would be to suggest that the special characteristics of human milk would make it better for calves. The milks are different because they have been created especially for the needs of the young of that species. Common sense would tell you that if human milk were fatally deficient, we wouldn't be here. We can trust our bodies to know more than our scientists. If our babies were supposed to be eating vegetables from birth, as some animals do, we would not be making milk at all. We would have more young, like turtles for example, many of whom die, instead of our usual one that is designed to live until maturity. It is a survival tactic that is very successful.

Formula has been so altered that it is like no animal's milk, and the way it differs from all mammal's milk is that it is not alive. It does not react to its recipient; to produce antibodies to a baby's infection for example, or change the amount of fat or water to the baby's taste or thirst as a mother's milk does. However we manipulate the ingredients in the factory, it is still a processed food that is far removed from the fresh product produced at source, on demand for the particular infants' needs.

The deficiencies in formula only come to light when babies become ill, and fail to thrive. There isn't any other way to find out. As I said, the needs of human infants are unique. The breast is already able to produce the ideal food for each baby.

Protection of breastmilk

Human milk contains a host of protective substances. The nutritional composition also supports the health of the infant by providing the ideal balance of nutrients for the infant, at the same time denying any dangerous organisms the chance to multiply. This is done by providing the minimum amount of iron, for example and binding it in such a way that the baby can utilize it (lactoferrin), but not any harmful bacteria that are present in the gut. There are other bacteria that humans find it useful to colonize the gut but they do not use iron. There are a number of sugars produced in human milk which remain undigested and appear to be present to inhibit the growth of dangerous organisms. There are the antibodies to all the diseases with which the mother has come into contact and to diseases that only the baby has met.

Here are some of the conditions that we know breastfeeding helps to prevent:

Constipation

Eczema

Asthma

Gastrointestinal infections

Respiratory infections

Urinary tract infections

Ear infections

Sudden infant death

Diabetes

Dental malocclusion

Childhood lymphoma

Bowel disease

Heart disease

Auto immune thyroid disease

Crohn's disease

Coeliac disease

Neonatal tetany

Multiple sclerosis

Appendicitis

Neonatal Necrotising Enterocolitis (in preterm infants)

Breastfeeding enhances immunity and increases intelligence in preterm and full term babies.

If a formula fed baby has gastroenteritis it is not necessarily because the mother has been careless in preparing the baby's feeds. It can be because cow's milk formula is not suited to human infants. The chance for error is always there though, from contaminated formula as well as non-sterile preparation. Protective mechanisms do exist in cow's milk too; they are either destroyed in the manufacturing process or unsuitable for human infants. The milk is, after all, designed for calves. This design includes encouraging the growth of bacteria to assist in the breakdown of grass, the cow's staple diet, and which are dangerous to human infants. So the very nature of the milk is designed to produce the conditions that are dangerous to babies. The opposite conditions from those provided by human milk (see *Breastfeeding Matters* and *The Politics of Breastfeeding*).

EXPECTATIONS

We all have expectations about breastfeeding. We may not know we do, indeed we may think that we do not, but they are there. If we did not have expectations we could never be disappointed. Our breastfeeding expectations may be that it is, or should be like formula feeding, if that is all we know. Or it may be that it is normal and natural if we have seen it many times before. Few people brought up in this country have an untainted view; it is hard to imagine anyone being exposed to open, unrestricted breastfeeding in our culture, and seeing it as the norm. Those couples I speak to who have been brought up in other cultures find it hard to believe that we have a problem with breastfeeding when they have seen it working well. Even so they may experience the problems that come with being isolated in a society that does not support a mother breastfeeding. The very reason why they could not see how breastfeeding could be difficult may be that they did not realize how supportive their culture was, and how important that support is to successful breastfeeding. When that support is absent, parents are without the knowledge they need from experienced people who know about managing breastfeeding well. If they experience problems themselves the advice they receive may not be compatible with continuing breastfeeding and they may not know why it has failed. The practice of giving 'supplementary' feeds to newborns to 'increase their weight gain' is a good case in point. First of all it suggests that the mother cannot make enough milk when she is new to breastfeeding. Then it suggests that her baby should be gaining more weight than it is. Finally the practice undermines the mother's milk supply just as she starts out, and she will end up not making enough if she continues to give formula.

You may not know that a normal breastfed baby's stool is bright yellow and runny. Breastfed babies absorb almost everything in their mother's milk, the yellow colouring comes from the bile used in the process of digestion, there is not much left to be passed in a motion. Some people worry that their baby is ill if they do not know that this is normal. Also, some breastfed babies only dirty a nappy every few days, others at every feed.

Birth Experience

The way a woman gives birth makes a big difference to her experience of initiating breastfeeding. If the birth is straightforward, mother and baby will be alert and responsive to one another, and this is the ideal time to learn about breastfeeding together. The feeling of elation after birth seems to be referred to little, though I have experienced it myself and have friends who have too. I spoke to the husband of one friend after a home birth and he said "She's in her usual state of postnatal euphoria". This contrasts with many women's experience of birth and explains why breastfeeding sometimes does not get off to a good start. Do not despair. If your birth is not everything you had hoped for you may find that breastfeeding gives you great satisfaction and restores your self confidence. The same is true of mothers who failed to breastfeed in the way that they would have liked to and yet go on to succeed with subsequent children. There is a spin off effect that helps to make up for the time before and improves your relationship with the previous child. Second- or subsequent-time mothers, who have bottle fed the first time, feel like first time mothers when it comes to breastfeeding and may find that everyone expects them to know what they are doing. You may have to ask for help.

Obviously if the mother is very tired after the birth she may just wish to sleep. Nature prepares the baby for this; he has enough fat stored to keep him going for several days while his mother recovers. During this time it is helpful if you can avoid giving the baby bottles of formula. This is something that fathers can explain if their partners are feeling weak; they can also put the baby to the mother's breast while she rests. The baby may be equally sleepy and uninterested in feeding until the mother feels stronger anyhow. Being born is tiring for the baby too. A new baby only needs a little breast milk each time he suckles to keep him going until both he and his mother have recovered.

If the mother has had drugs during delivery this can make an enormous difference to the responsiveness of the baby. The effect may take a week to wear off. If the baby is born by Caesarean section, breastfeeding is still possible, though the mother will need physical assistance. I cover Caesarean section in Special

Circumstances p.148.

Women who have home births find breastfeeding easier to initiate. They have privacy, only a few chosen people around and their familiar surroundings. Those women who feel safer giving birth in hospital sometimes choose to go home early to breastfeed in peace. For a first baby, some women like to be in hospital where they feel more help is at hand. Whatever your situation, keep asking until you get the help you need and don't feel that all is lost if you do not get off to the ideal start you had planned. You have about 4 weeks to play with while you and your baby learn about each other, and during this time you may have to make several attempts at establishing breastfeeding, before you are up and running.

Afterpains

While breastfeeding the womb contracts after delivery and continues to do so for a couple of days. This is caused by the same hormone, oxytocin, that squeezes the milk sacs during let down. These contractions can be really strong, making it difficult to relax while you nurse. They can be just as powerful with a first baby, as I discovered after being told that they only affected you after subsequent babies... It is a small comfort to know that it is good for your body that your womb is contracting well and it means that everything is working properly.

How to avoid problems

If possible follow these suggestions. If you cannot, do not panic, you can start again when you feel better or once you get home.

Offer the breast as soon as possible after the birth, within one hour if possible.
Be patient, he may not latch on quickly.
Do not offer bottles.
Feed frequently at first, every hour or as often as he will nurse (some will simply sleep).
Leave him on the breast until he comes off himself.
Trust him to know how much he wants.
Trust your body to make what he needs.
Encourage your baby to feed if you feel full.
Keep your baby with you, hold him as much as you like.
Do not continue to nurse if you are in pain, find

someone to help you latch him on better.

Make sure you are looked after as well as the baby.

Allow people to look after you, do the washing up, make tea while you look after the baby.

Don't feel you have to be perfect.

Find support.

Get ready for a feed, have a drink near you, book for toddler, potty etc.

Learn to nurse lying down.

Personality of the baby

A major consideration in the course of breastfeeding your baby is his personality. This seems to be generally overlooked. Babies are considered to be much the same when they are young. I have found this not to be the case. When dealing with particular couples I notice how the mother and baby interact, the personality of the baby is as large a determinant in the relationship as the mother's. This is particularly noticeable in a mother who has been in touch with me before about a previous baby. One mother contacted me about her second baby; she had thought breastfeeding this time around would be straightforward since she had solved the problem with her first child and gone on to nurse for fifteen months. She had not reckoned with the impatient nature of her second baby, who refused to nurse at all if her mother was not quick enough to latch her on the first time she asked.

Different ideas and techniques are required for different mother and baby couples.

The individuality of the baby also seems to be a large determinant in the length and frequency of feeds. Some people associate a large baby with being 'a hungry baby' meaning that he feeds a lot, other people assume that a large baby will be able to go longer between feeds because he is bigger. I have not noticed such a direct connection with size. Anyway some people's idea of a large baby is a small one to another, and they all grow to be a lot bigger and still breastfed if you keep at it. So a large baby at birth is obviously not going to be as big as a fully breastfed six month old, and it is quite possible to breastfeed whatever the size of the baby.

A problem does arise, however, when a woman expects breastfeeding to be difficult and does not make a fuss when the demands upon her are completely unreasonable. There may be something wrong that needs attending to. A mother rang me recently whose baby never slept for longer than 20 minutes and was crying a lot at night. She mentioned that she had changed to decaffeinated coffee when her baby was young, but was now drinking ordinary coffee again some months later. She was understandably exhausted. Babies are affected by the mother drinking coffee – even decaffeinated may affect the baby. This baby was obviously not happy, and this is the guideline as to whether your baby is behaving normally. If you can tell that he is really tired but cannot sleep, or sleeps fitfully, look for what may be causing the problem. See also Crying and Colic p.139 and p.142.

Questions – Preparing each other

I suggest to couples before their baby is born that they ask each other some questions about their baby being breastfed. The idea behind this is that you have found out before a moment of crisis what each of you was expecting and may therefore be able to avoid a heated argument at a stressful time. Think about each question individually for a moment and then share your feeling about what may be appropriate for you. For example, it is really helpful to know if your partner will be expecting your baby to be fed in private every time visitors come around after the birth. This can be practically impossible if the mother wants to see anything of the visitors and the baby feeds erratically - as most newborns do. However it would be fine if you both agreed about it and arranged what to do about the visitors.

The questions I suggest are:

For how long would you like your baby to be breastfed?
Where would you be happy for your baby to be breastfed?
In front of whom would you feel comfortable when your baby is being breastfed?
These are the questions I ask in an antenatal class. You could also ask:
Where are you expecting your baby to sleep at night?
What will you do if you find through circumstances beyond your control that soon after birth your baby is being formula fed?
How willing are you to question what is being done to your baby by other people?

At what point would you ask for help? from a breastfeeding counsellor perhaps.

You may not have answers to all of these, but the process of having discussed them will have given you an idea of how your partner feels about these issues, and how much you can ask of each other and rely on them for support.

There are a wide variety of answers to these questions. They are personal issues. The problem can arise when each person thinks that the way they feel is the only way it should be done. That's why it is good to air them before the baby arrives and you can make plans. Of course people change their minds. The two issues that strike me most are sleeping arrangements and nursing in public. Those parents who are adamant that their baby will not sleep in their bed or nurse in public are often the ones who end up doing so because the baby needs to. This is why I tell people about these things: so that they are aware that they have a choice. If you know what is possible you can make the appropriate decision at the time. Also breastfeeding lasts longer than the birth, so even if things do not go according to plan you can try again later. It is useful to make known your wishes about breastfeeding to your health carers.

Clocks

There is no place for timing in a full term healthy breastfed baby's feeding. Many of the problems experienced by breastfeeding couples stem from eagerness to regulate. The fashion for this is dying out but there remains a fear of overindulgence if a baby's' needs are met consistently. In fact the production of the milk relies on the baby taking what it needs. The system is adaptable enough to cater for each baby's preferences producing the amount, type and consistency at different times of the day and throughout each feed. It is also flexible enough to meet a baby's increasing demands as it grows or when it is unwell within a matter of hours, given adequate access to the breast.
Most babies do, however, develop a pattern of their own. This may take several weeks to establish. It will also change every few weeks as the baby grows and needs to stimulate the breast further to increase production. It also changes if baby or mother are ill.
We have been led to believe that babies feed at regular

intervals. For example every 2 or 3 hours. They may not any more than adults do. Since they have smaller stomachs they can be expected to eat a lot more frequently than adults eat. Babies, also like adults, vary enormously in the length of time they are prepared to go without food.

Mothers who do not wish to feed their babies in public find it useful to learn this pattern in order to organise activities around it. Some babies are predictable in this way, but a lot aren't. If you have one that isn't, I include some suggestions of how to deal with the situation in which you find yourself and still have a life (see Discreet Nursing p.77).

The difference in feeding times between normal babies is illustrated beautifully by two of my children who were of a similar weight at birth and put on about the same amount each week. The first of my daughters fed for an hour every two hours, the other fed for one and a half minutes every hour and a half (on one side only per feed). This took me by surprise after the first one! It shows how different two babies can be, even in the same family and with the same parents. The breasts adjust to the different feeding patterns of each baby. This second baby was born during a hot summer and began nursing on two breasts each feed many months later. I also fed her on one side during the day and the other at night because it was convenient to me to use my right hand for other things while feeding in the day – and nurse on the left side.

Fortunately it is no longer fashionable to expect babies to go for four hours between feeds. Some people do still remember this as a figure to aim for however, and to them I would say that in the fourteen years I have been dealing with mothers and babies I recall only two babies that have fed regularly every four hours by choice. There is nothing to be gained by trying to get a baby to feed less frequently just for the sake of it. If we want our children healthier and breastfed, then we need to make the information available about what is normal in breastfeeding, so parents know what to expect. At present some mothers are choosing to formula feed because they do not want to feed their babies as frequently as they see breastfeeding needing to be done. This is only a problem if it cramps the mother's lifestyle, and I would love to see it become more acceptable for women to nurse their babies wherever they were, and not formula feed because they feel it is more convenient. Physically it is easier to breastfeed; there is no preparation needed, no washing of bottles and teats, no need to buy formula. So the pressure against breastfeeding must be enormous for women to voluntarily take on this burden. If we could change our perspective on the difficulty and undesirability of breastfeeding, it would seem the easier option and women would choose to do it.

Babies need for sleep – sleeping arrangements

All mammals sleep with their young. Most humans do as well. It is only here in Britain and the USA that a notion has arisen that babies can be expected to sleep alone. This is relevant to breastfeeding because you are then not expected to wake in the night to nurse your baby. An ideal baby, according to society, is one that sleeps all night alone. It is not surprising that parents become exhausted and possibly resentful about this, and they are unprepared, when they discover the reality that their baby needs attention during the night.

I talked to a Chinese woman who had never been to Europe about the British habit of leaving babies alone to sleep when very young and she said "But the baby would be scared!". She was genuinely shocked at the idea.

Interestingly in a survey reported in our local paper in Solihull last year 66% of parents questioned said they would allow a child into their bed when unwell.

I know many parents here do sleep with their babies. They rarely talk about it though, which means that other parents don't think it is normal and OK, and they struggle on unsupported.

If you know that is what a baby will expect you don't have such a shock when your brand new baby cries when put down alone. I say this so that you know what to expect and that you are not doing anything wrong if your baby does not obediently drop off in its own room as portrayed so convincingly in the advertising we see in this country. The practice of expectant parents preparing a room for their baby before it is born speaks for itself, showing the expectation of our culture that a new baby is instantly ready to be separate from its mother. Appropriately this room is called a Nursery – from the nurse who used to be available to the baby all the time by those who paid someone else to look after their baby and yes, you've guessed, to sleep beside it.

Breastfeeding needs proximity and certainly for the first few months (or longer if you plan to continue nursing) you can expect a baby to need to feed in the night. If you know that this is normal behaviour you won't worry when it happens to you. I hope it will also prevent you from spending many fruitless hours pacing the floor in the small hours with a baby who sleeps soundly while you are holding it and wakes like magic as soon as it is put down and you attempt to leave the room.

This is a safety mechanism in the baby to know when you are near and it is being protected. We are still biologically the same animals that have survived in the wild. And, as stated by Jean Liedloff in the 'Continuum Concept', there are still places in the world where your baby would be eaten by a leopard if left alone. Our babies cannot know that we don't live in the wilderness. The fact that our babies are more at threat from another human being than a wild animal is sad but means that we still need to be vigilant in protecting our young ones.

When I had my first baby I felt uneasy about going out of the room without her. My neighbour expressed the same feeling in hospital and was laughed at. However since recent baby snatching incidents she feels that she has a right to be protective.

All this is not to say that you should or should not do things a particular way, but in order that you might know what to expect and what is possible. Some babies do sleep in a room alone, some parents have the baby in the same room and some in a crib beside the bed. All of these can work, as can putting the baby down alone for the first part of the night then bringing it into your bed for the rest of the night. This solution can give you the best of both worlds. You only have to wake once, you get the privacy and relaxation of going to bed alone / with your partner, the baby sleeps most soundly for the first few hours as you do, breastfeeding can then continue for the rest of the night without you being woken. This or something similar can work, then it changes as the baby matures. Sometimes the new baby does need to be held all the time and you can try this once some weeks have passed. You have to be creative in finding ways to get the most sleep for everyone in the most acceptable manner. Some mothers have a single bed in the baby's room that they go to after the baby wakes to save disturbing their partner and to give them more room. Some people get a bigger bed. I had a single bed by our double bed once my second baby was seven months old so she could crawl in with me when she needed to, I did not then have to wake at all.

It all changes in time and children do move on to the next stage when ready.

A description of sleeping with a baby

Some parents sleep with the baby between them. Others put the baby on the mother's side, the mother sleeps on her side and feeds the baby in this position. I found that feeding from either breast while lying on the same side saved disturbance and could be done by tilting my body. One of my children only fed on one side in the night and on the other during the day – this shows the flexibility of the system. The breasts will adjust to whatever is demanded of them in time, amount and type of milk to be produced. I had two pillows and tucked my shoulder up to them, putting my lower arm around the baby. You also need something – or someone – to support your back so you can relax completely and sleep.

I also wrapped a little sheet around the baby when

small and tucked it under me because I was worried about her falling onto the floor. She never did. Later I had a single bed next to ours; you can also put a pillow on the floor.

There is a story about an African midwife being asked about how the mothers know where their babies are when they are asleep with them, and she replied that you know where the edge of the bed is and don't fall out in the night, even when you are fast asleep.

I first considered the idea of sleeping with my second baby after an exhausting time with a first baby who was not happy sleeping alone. I couldn't face the idea of being kept awake with a crying baby for most of the night and having a lively toddler to look after all day. It just was not sensible; so after a period of thinking that perhaps an only child was the best solution... I planned to tuck the next one down under the quilt beside me and see if it worked. I tried when I had my three day old in my own bed for the first time. The feeling of joy and delight at my success when I woke up feeling rested at 6.45 the next morning has never left me! She had fed about six times in the night but I was barely aware of it. I understand that if you are awake for less than fifteen seconds it doesn't disturb your sleep. It only takes a moment to latch a little one on and they soon get the hang of doing it for themselves. If they are down under the quilt beside you, you leave a gap for the air to reach them and they will probably not need to wear anything other than a nappy.

I discovered to my delight at this time that my baby didn't soil a nappy if not fully wakened to feed. She merely stirred in her sleep and fed without ever opening her eyes. She was a bit soggy in the morning and so needed an extra absorbent nappy for night. While breastfeeding you may need to protect the bed from milk leaking - with a folded terry nappy or towel.

The problem I am usually faced with when a baby apparently won't sleep is the exhaustion of the parents. Babies can sleep anywhere anytime and the adults need to be considered.   It is useful to know that breastfeeding reduces the mother's need for sleep and cuts out the deepest stage of sleep altogether. This means that you are always conscious of where your baby is and able to respond. This mechanism is not reliable, however, if you take sleeping tablets or large quantities of alcohol. It also doesn't exist if you are bottle feeding – 'though many bottle feeding parents do sleep with their babies too. Michel Odent (author of "Birth Reborn" and pioneer of water birth) noticed when he visited eastern countries, where bottle feeding is rapidly replacing breastfeeding, that parents still universally sleep with their babies.

The problem can be the parents' acceptance of the idea of sharing their bed with their baby. Some couples are delighted with the idea and readily take to the peaceful system it can provide. Others resist the idea and may only try it in desperation, their motivation being to get a quiet night, but not feeling comfortable with it. You need to discuss this. Some people worry about rolling onto the baby. This fear has arisen from the practice of Victorian wet nurses deliberately suffocating their own new born babies so that they could nurse others and earn a living. They told the authorities that they had lain on them by mistake. Clearly those in authority did not look after their own babies as they believed the story. I had an experience with one of my babies, aged six weeks, who ended up in between her dad and I – I don't know how she got there – and when he turned over onto her she poked him with her little knees and elbows and shouted until he woke up.

Not all newborns need to sleep all the time that they are not feeding. I feel that as long as the baby is content there is no need to be concerned about whether or not it is sleeping. Parents' sleep seems to be much more precious to me. The disturbance of their sleep, if it is causing distress, is more important than the baby's since it can sleep anytime, anywhere.

Some newborn babies do sleep all day and all night. This seems quite common for the first two days – even in babies whose mothers have received no drugs during labour which can cause an abnormally sleepy baby that is difficult to feed for several days. After this, normal sleep variation is enormous. Some need only half an hour in the day. My daughter, then three, was surprised that her baby brother should sleep at all during the day. She obviously had not read the right childcare books. He was one of those who only slept for half an hour or so. Since he was completely content to watch us and be carried about the rest of the time it really didn't matter.

I think it is useful to remember that this phase will not last forever, our children will sleep through the night when they are older. Some take a long time, but they all do it. I would also like to point out that since adults choose to be awake during the night for many recreational reasons, I consider it quite reasonable to attend to your little ones during the night, and justify this to anyone who might criticize you.

Toddler nursing

Some parents have a definite idea of how long their children will be breastfed, others have not decided or change their minds after they have begun.

Culturally, the expectation here appears to suggest that breastfeeding is something that you might do for a while before you begin giving bottles of formula. At any rate sometime your baby will be getting a bottle surely …

To continue to breastfeed solely until your child is eating many nourishing other foods is unusual, and to continue long after it is deemed necessary, is often seen as self indulgence on the part of the mother. The parents who continue realize the benefits to their child in nourishment, protection and security and they listen to what their child has to say. By the time some children are ready to give up nursing they are indeed able to say what they want. It is wonderful to hear your child telling you how much he appreciates nursing.

I remember when I was nursing a toddler of my own – about 16 months old – seeing a friend nursing her child and he was wearing shoes. It struck me that it was a strange sight to see someone else nursing a toddler even though I was doing so myself.

Toddlers continue to nurse for the benefits of nutrition, bearing in mind that they may eat fairly erratically; for comfort, when they have fallen over or been upset; when they are tired, many nurslings continue only the night time feed for many months; and when they are ill, in which case they may go back to fully nursing and you will be surprised to find yourself making pints of milk again after the quantity had been slowly diminishing. This latter reason is so convenient for the parents, as it ensures that the child is not dangerously ill, and often means that you do not have to resort to medication. I liked the fact that I did not have to sit awake at night with ill children as long as they could nurse.

One of the problems that faces the parents of nursing toddlers is that if they have any difficulty that they are dealing with, it is attributed to the fact that they are still nursing. Some problems are made different by the fact that you are still nursing, and have to be handled bearing that in mind. But most are unrelated and affect many children at that stage (useful book "Mothering your nursing toddler").

You may begin to get remarks about weaning when your baby is only a few months old. It depends on where you live and who else you know who is breastfeeding. It is comforting to join a breastfeeding group for moral support while you are breastfeeding. I found it extremely helpful. I also made some really good friends, who have remained long after our children have stopped nursing. This is the sort of support that is wonderful when you are nursing your child and you know that it is right for you to continue. It helps when the doubts creep in, as most of our families and neighbours will not be doing or believing in the same thing (see breastfeeding groups, useful addresses: Association of Breastfeeding Mothers, La Leche League, also the National Childbirth Trust has a Breastfeeding Promotion Group and some breastfeeding mothers support groups).
Once you have been nursing for more than nine months or a year, you may come under some extraordinary pressure to stop nursing. Some people find it even

more offensive to see an older child nurse. At this point some women then choose only to nurse at home. This can work quite well, as an eighteen month old for example, can understand 'when we get home'. Having said that I feel that our children's welfare is more important than the uninvited disapproval of strangers so sometimes we may have to risk criticism while we attend to our own child's' needs.

A visit to a breastfeeding country is a refreshing break, worth remembering if you are planning to go away with your family. It is so supportive to see all the women publicly feeding their children and reminds us that it is our society that is being odd, not us.

Weaning

This term means the introduction of food other than breastmilk. It does not mean that the baby stops nursing. The overlap of breastfeeding and eating other foods is meant to be a large safety margin. The longer a child receives breastmilk the healthier he will be. The benefits are measurable way beyond infancy. I am saying this because it appears that in this country it is assumed that once a baby has solid food it will no longer need milk. It also appears to be a cause for pride to have a child who is precociously mature, having 'solid food' – which is in fact liquefied food – at only a few weeks that its gut is not ready to receive. The child is not ready until it is able to chew at least a little with its gums, if not teeth, and need never have pureed food at all. This readiness happens somewhere in the middle of the first year and may be related to when your baby cuts his teeth. Some are not ready for many months, even up to a year. Formula fed babies must receive other foods because formula is known not to be a perfect food for infants. This knowledge has then been transferred to breastfed babies because of fears about the inadequacy of milk. It does not apply to breastmilk in the same way and it is perfectly appropriate to feed a baby solely on breastmilk for at least six months. At about this time most babies will have started to show an interest in the food that you are eating. I found that my babies liked to nurse when we were having a meal, so it was natural for them to share as much as they could manage. I did have to draw the line at one daughter who used to nurse avidly and eat half the food off my plate. I thought it was time to give her her own meal.

Many parents assume that babies need pureed food to begin with and even that it must be especially bought in little jars. Of course you can give your baby these foods if you wish but you do not need to. By starting your child on what you eat the chance is that he will continue to eat the same food as you with little fuss. When your baby stretches out his hand to try your food he wants what you are eating, not what you have separately prepared or bought. Once ready, a baby can manage to gnaw and suck at anything it can hold:

 crusts of toast

 quarters of apple

 peas

 chunks of banana

 dried apricots and figs

these will keep a baby happily occupied for ages. You can also pass spoons of mashed potato, rice, sauces from your plate. A baby sitting and chewing may choke, so you need to be ready to tip them up over the sink if necessary, and they should always be attended. Stopping nursing is a different matter from introducing other foods. This can cause heated debate, and is one topic I suggest you discuss with your partner, before you begin if possible.

Any breastmilk is better than none, so do begin, whatever your later plans. The colostrum, first milk, is highly protective and lines the baby's gut ready to receive mature milk. You need to nurse for a minimum of seventeen weeks if you wish to protect your baby from the more damaging effects of respiratory disease and gastroenteritis. However I would guess that if you get that far you are unlikely to want to change as you have got through the tricky bit and onto the enjoyable part. It is after all a wonderful experience to nurse your baby and not just a matter of the best feeding method. Many people assume that breastfeeding will be halted by a mother's return to work. This is not the case. Do plan to breastfeed, even if you feel you later will be returning to work. Mothers who go out to work often continue to breastfeed and really value the relationship they have through continued nursing. You can continue to nurse morning and evening for many months, and this has a protective function as well as an emotional bond. (see Work: returning to work and breastfeeding p.150, and the book *Working and Breastfeeding*)

The ideal is to let the child choose how long to nurse,

if that is what you would like to do. Most will choose to stop when over one year old. In many countries, and in some religions, there are stipulations as to the least time you should nurse. There are also indications to stop so that the mother can conceive again. The World Health Organisation recommends at least two years, in industrialized nations as well as in countries where the child's health is more obviously at risk. It is becoming more widely recognized that breastfeeding protects against infectious diseases – especially in areas without access to clean water. However it is less well known that formula fed babies are five times more likely to die than breastfed babies in this country (The UK). And here we notice the preventative effect of breastfeeding on diseases like childhood diabetes, asthma and ear infections.

If you have decided that you do wish to instigate the end of breastfeeding, plan to do it gradually, for your benefit as well as the baby's. Sudden weaning can cause painful engorgement, even when you thought that your milk supply had dwindled.

Suggestions of times not to wean (terminate breastfeeding): when baby or mother are unwell, when you are about to move house or go on holiday, because someone in authority disapproves of the age of your nursling, when the next baby comes if you are still nursing, during a heatwave. These times may precipitate your need to reconsider your relationship with your child and partner but they can be a mistaken time to force weaning if everything just seems too much. At stressful times it can be disheartening to find your nursling apparently regressing by getting more enthusiastic about breastfeeding. It is temporary. Parents tell me they notice that their children are more independent than their contemporaries, when they have chosen to wean themselves from the breast in their own time. However there are times of natural maturing and some children decide that they will wean themselves at significant moments; there are no rules.

PRACTICALITIES

How to avoid problems

Here are some suggestions. Do not worry if you cannot follow them all – women have begun to breastfeed later than they wanted to and still succeeded:

Clothing

I started off unbuttoning my clothes down the front with my first baby which was cold as well as indiscreet. Then I realized that if I lifted my shirt from the bottom I could keep all my top layers on and be unnoticed at the same time.

Whenever I ask a class of mixed couples who thinks that they are wearing suitable clothes for breastfeeding they look for ones that undo down the front. So I feel it is worth pointing out that the almost universal wear of sweatshirts and tee shirts is ideal for breastfeeding. You need clothes that you can lift up rather than undo down the front. The layers need to be fairly light and as my friend points out, no mohair: the baby gets all tangled in mouthfuls of the fluff.

There are companies specializing in smarter clothes with hidden zips. These can be useful and are easy to undo but may need assistance to do back up again (if a dress zip is in the side seam). Remember you may only have one hand to use as you are holding the baby. Another friend pointed out that it would be useful if the concealed zips in front darts or pockets undid from the bottom rather than the top for discreet nursing. It is harder to be discreet with fitted clothing so a shawl comes in handy if you find yourself breastfeeding at a wedding reception...

Bras

Much advice is given about the wearing of bras in pregnancy and while breastfeeding, and while many women find it more comfortable to wear one, there are advantages and disadvantages. The skin will change during pregnancy and I believe has more to do with diet than the wearing of a bra (particularly lack of vitamin E). I also think that the changes are a part of maturing that pregnancy brings. Our culture is unusual in its obsession with youthfulness and wanting to appear not to have had children. In other cultures motherhood is something to be proud of and the signs of childbearing are status symbols. The significance of the correct bra in this country during pregnancy – and even suggested during sleep – betrays the importance of warding off stretch marks or the sagging breast. I suspect that some changes are inevitable, and it is still possible to have a beautiful, lithe body, even if it has changed a little. Most other people will not notice, and usually partners of worried women whose bodies have changed still find them attractive – and may not even notice the difference that the woman is so conscious of.

Careful fitting of bras for breastfeeding is important as an ill-fitting bra can block the ducts which is painful and inconvenient. The style of bra needs to be looked at to see if one part of the breast is pressed while feeding (eg Trapdoor type). It is also good if you can find a style that you can undo with one hand.

Breast pads are often used to soak up leaking milk in bras. They prevent contact of air with the breast so it may be unwise to use them continuously. This can be a cause of sore nipples. Some women have found that the pressure of the bra is making them leak so they don't need the pads if they don't wear the bra. Leaking is much more common in the early days, so you may not find that you have to deal with the situation in public. Since breast size can change enormously in pregnancy and during breastfeeding the wearing of a bra is a personal choice about comfort and convenience. When your baby is very young and learning how to latch on, a bra often just gets in the way.

If you have trouble finding a nursing bra the National Childbirth Trust have a very wide range of fittings available and will help you ensure you have the size you need. While women are concerned about the correct bra when they begin breastfeeding, many find that once their breasts have become accustomed to producing milk, they can wear an ordinary bra. A low cut one is ideal for having access to the breast and is easy to pull aside and replace discreetly. I found that once I was regularly producing at a certain rate my bra size was a familiar 34B, despite the fact that the first flush of milk production had made me huge, and that later I must have been producing more milk for my much larger baby. This system works if the baby feeds frequently but comes unstuck if the baby sleeps for an unusually long stretch and the breasts fill to capacity. Avoid underwired bras, they are uncomfortable and the pressure on the breast can cause obstruction.

Nursing bras are almost always white. For those women who prefer active wear there are bras in brighter colours and sports designs (see useful addresses: Bravado bras).

Leaking

During the early days of breastfeeding it is common for the breasts to leak milk, especially when full. This is messy, but usually does not last. It does mean that you need to be prepared; for example during the night if your baby sleeps longer than expected, you can end up with a wet mattress unless you have a thick towel. Sleeping on one side often causes that side to leak. Once you have been nursing for some weeks, you generally find it subsides. Some women then worry that they are not then making as much milk. I suggest that leaking is more a 'valve' problem than a supply problem. It seems to happen more with one baby than another too – with the same mother.

If you press the heel of your hand briefly into the breast on the nipple as it lets down you can stop it from leaking. This is useful if you are nursing in public and do not want your clothes drenched. You can also do this with a finger. Be careful not to be overenthusiastic with this though to avoid damage such as blocked ducts. When in private you can catch the milk with a cloth as the baby latches onto the other breast and it lets down. It stops on its own.

Leaking can happen spontaneously during lovemaking too, not just from pressure, but because oxytocin – the hormone causing contractions of the womb during orgasm is also responsible for expressing milk from the breast during nursing. I am warning so you – and your partner – don't get a surprise. When you leak don't worry about wasting milk; only a proportion of foremilk comes out and it is soon replaced.

Sex

For some couples the chance to make love properly after months of the baby literally coming between them is a cause for celebration and something they are eager to enjoy. I loved the experience of freedom to be close after the bump disappeared with my second and third babies: I had an intact perineum and felt wonderful! Breastfeeding need not make a difference to your sex life, although you will probably leak milk as I have already mentioned (See leaking above). Making love as soon as you feel ready maintains your feeling special for each other despite the changes a new baby brings. Some first time parents are so overwhelmed by the birth, their new status and the woman's painful stitches – which she did not expect and are rather a shock – to worry about breastfeeding interfering with sex. Later though (and it may be months later), when they want to reestablish their physical intimacy, it is worth having considered what differences there will be. The longer the gap, the more of an issue it may become.

The baby's unscheduled feeding times and the woman's changed body shape and function can make the experience a bit like the first time over again. Stitches are painful: if you continue to have a problem make sure you get it seen to, rather than use the excuse of the baby waking to avoid sex, if you are worried about pain. Talk about it.

Your breastfeeding baby can be less of an intrusion than a bottle fed one because you can nurse him immediately and then he need not fully waken.

Discreet Nursing

The idea of nursing your baby in public can be a bit daunting.

Try:

Practising in front of a mirror

Taking a shawl – to put around you and the baby

Not looking people in the eye in a public place

On a bus or train, take a window seat and face the window while nursing

Feeding the baby BEFORE he cries and draws attention to you

It is sad that we feel we have to cover ourselves while breastfeeding, but if we want to feel as relaxed as possible I reckon it's worth the effort of not antagonising if we can. Having said that I feel that if we are discreet then we should be able to nurse anywhere. This is the society we live in so let's deal with it how it is while we work on how we would like it to be.

Some people will notice whatever you do. These are usually mothers who have breastfed themselves, know the tell tale signs like gulping noises, and are really supportive. Children will want to know what you are doing. Be prepared for the probing questions of the children of bottle-feeding mothers. They will ask what you are doing and when you tell them they will look disbelievingly and ask where the bottle is. A survey of Scottish children recently discovered that a proportion of them do not know that people are mammals.

Carrying your baby while nursing can be an answer to the busy mother who has a baby who likes to constantly nurse. Wrapping a baby Welsh fashion in a shawl was shown to me when I had my third child and I found it useful. You can do almost anything while wearing it because it leaves both hands free. The women used to work in the mines wearing them! You need a big shawl, folded diagonally. You hold the baby in one arm, wrap the shawl around both shoulders, wrap one end right over the baby and tuck it under your arm and the baby, the other shorter end you pull tight and push under the same arm, using the weight of the baby to keep it in place. Like this, you have one arm free and one hand free. The woman who showed me demonstrated how she could cook while carrying her baby. The shawl is a lovely way to carry a child while you are outside, especially if the child is feeling unwell. An antenatal teacher I have worked with recalls being carried Welsh fashion by her mother until she was about two.

There are also some baby carriers that it is possible to discreetly nurse in, the La Leche League supply a selection of types.

I find it fascinating though to learn that in some countries where the women cover their heads and their bodies in public they can expose their breast to feed their baby. It shows how cultures vary. It wasn't always so in this country either. Until 1945 women openly breastfed on trains in front of strangers.

Diet

This is a time when it is useful to eat well: your body has undergone enormous changes after supporting your growing child for nine months, you are now in a novel situation for which you probably have had little useful preparation, and you may be getting very little sleep. It is therefore a time when you will be unlikely to feel able to do much about your diet. If you have supportive relatives who genuinely want to be helpful. Get them to feed you.

When I had my first child, I was awake too often for too long, and felt that the demands upon me were overwhelming. There was practically no way that I could resolve my situation. At this time I came across Adele Davis' book on nutrition and found a useful idea. She suggested fortifying foods for combatting exhaustion, I used some of her ideas to good effect and have since developed an interest in promoting health through nutrition as well as for preventing specific disorders.

A woman can breastfeed whatever her diet; however the mother herself may suffer if her diet is woefully inadequate. Her baby will get a balanced diet from her milk. The quality of breast milk is extraordinarily consistent despite enormous differences in the amount and type of food intake of different women. As in pregnancy a woman's gut works more efficiently while she is nursing. Generally people only use a proportion of the nutrients that they eat. You will probably find that you are very hungry – I used to get through a whole loaf of wholemeal bread a day when nursing my bonny babies. It is a perk of breastfeeding to be able to eat and enjoy more food than usual.

'Everything in moderation' is a useful guideline for what to eat when breastfeeding. Do not cut out foods that other women have had problems with unless they cause a problem for your baby. Some women restrict their diet just in case their baby has a problem. This is unnecessary and may cause a deficiency itself. You can, however, be aware of certain foods that commonly cause problems if your baby is habitually distressed, as these may be the first to investigate. Cow's milk protein, egg, certain fruits and green vegetables have all been known to cause problems. See Crying and Colic p.139 and p.142 if you need to follow this up. A mother I knew ate a whole loaf of new bread out of a batch she had just baked when her baby was young, and the baby complained. I think it was just too much of one thing. Another mother was given some grapes and plums – she ate them all – no one had told her that it could be a mistake. Her poor baby lay without a nappy for several days while his skin recovered. The fruit had made his urine so acidic that his skin was raw.

The greatest increase in need during breastfeeding is for unrefined carbohydrate.
This is plentiful in whole foods: wholemeal bread flour

(preferably stone ground as it preserves vitamin E, see below) and wholemeal pasta, wholegrain rice, potatoes with skins on, root vegetables, fruit – bananas and avocados are energy rich but all fruit has useful sugar, peanut butter, dried fruit, fresh nuts and seeds. Snacks of these last few are some of the easiest ways to get nutritious food when you are on the run. It seems extraordinary that there are not enough hours in the day while your baby is young to eat a satisfying meal or have an uninterrupted bath. It feels claustrophobic sometimes and I understand why parents end up eating convenience foods that are not nutritious. Don't worry if this happens. Just get some useful food and eat it as well later. A combination of ready made foods and fresh fruit or salad will get you through the early days very well. A mother I met ate peanut butter and banana sandwiches while she breastfed, nutritionally quite sound. We worry that food is not as nutritious if it is not in the form of a proper meal. Although it is sometimes nice to sit down and eat together, making sure that your snack meals in the meantime are nutritious is a realistic approach.

The most useful drink is water.

Other drinks, especially stimulants like coffee and tea,

can cause fretful babies if taken in greater quantities than your baby can tolerate. Do not think that fruit juices are harmless, the amount in one orange juice for example is the same as eating perhaps ten oranges which you would never do, your baby may get a sore bottom from acidic urine. Some mothers tell me that they do not like drinking water and they have very diluted fruit drinks instead. You will probably find that you feel thirsty just as you begin to nurse your baby. I discovered that if I leave a jug of water to stand the chlorine bubbles up out of it and it tastes much nicer.

There is no need to avoid alcohol in the same way as is recommended while pregnant. Stout is suggested for nursing mothers because of the B vitamins it contains, only drink it if you like it though. Alcohol does go through into the milk, as does everything you eat, and may make your baby sleepy. Obviously it is recommended that you drink in moderation. Mothers ask if it is alright to have wine with a meal or champagne at a wedding, and the answer is yes.

The need for protein is easily covered by the foods already mentioned for energy.

Breastmilk contains about 1% protein which is all that human infants need.

B Vitamins are important in producing milk and are removed in the process of refining foods. So eat wholemeal bread etc. as mentioned above. Yeast extract is a good source (Marmite), some vegetarian margarines have them added.

Vitamin C is needed as it is present in breast milk. It enables the body to fight infections and is needed to absorb iron. Fresh food each day, even if it is an apple eaten as a snack is valuable. Fruit is an easy food to eat, with no preparation involved; eat a variety if you can.

Vitamin E is used by the body to keep the skin supple and reduce inflammation. It is essential in the development of the embryo too so a great deal is used in pregnancy. It is also deficient in the standard diet. One estimate I have seen suggests that since we have started processing flour, during which the wheat germ is discarded (eg white bread, breakfast cereals) our intake has gone from 150 to 7.4 units a day. It is present in nuts, seeds and grains – in the oil – so you can get it in cold pressed oils to put on salads. I also put oil on pasta and baked potatoes. Another easy way to increase your intake is to add some wheat germ to your breakfast. The problem is that vitamin E is destroyed by heating and storage, so most of the foods we eat have either been treated in such a way to destroy most of it or stored so long that it is no longer useful. The tell tale sign of staleness is the bitter taste, for example in nuts. As a child I thought nuts were horrid bitter things until I tasted fresh ones and discovered that nuts may have been stored for up to three years before we buy them.

Calcium is present in many foods and its absorption is complicated. It is not well absorbed by humans from cow's milk so vegetable sources may be better. Eating more of it does not necessarily increase absorption. Other factors are more important, for example making sure that vitamin D is present. A diet rich in unrefined foods will ensure that enough calcium is available, and daylight on the skin will ensure enough vitamin D, as it can be stored. If you are worried about vitamin D intake, maybe you have dark skin for example, you will find that the fortified foods available for vegetarians often have it added. Seeds are a good source of calcium, sunflower, pumpkin, sesame (tahini), nuts, beans and peas. Molasses is a rich food source – of calcium, iron, B vitamins – and is a useful sandwich filling.

I am not trying to create a comprehensive list here, but to cover the subjects of the questions most frequently asked about diet with breastfeeding.

Teeth

People sometimes assume that you will give up breastfeeding when your baby gets teeth. I had no intention of doing so as I knew that babies could cut their teeth at a few months, and I planned to breastfeed for a year. As it turned out my babies did cut their teeth early – at 3 and 4 months – but we continued to nurse happily. If a baby is going to bite he may well do so before he has teeth, as this is when the need to chew is greatest, before the tooth breaks through the gum. He has all his teeth in his gums already, so you may need to put your finger quickly between his jaws if he begins to hurt you.

The baby does not bite during the process of feeding because his tongue is between his teeth and your breast. The milk is not expressed by a biting action, it is obtained by rolling the tongue and bottom jaw together. Some mothers do have trouble with biting at the breast when their babies cut teeth. The natural reaction to getting bitten is to yelp or jump, and that sometimes does the trick and the baby does not bite again. Alternatively you can remove him from the breast and say "NO" firmly. (Take the baby off by putting your little finger in the corner of his mouth to break the suction.) Sometimes the baby starts to chew the breast at the end of the feed and the best thing to do is to keep watch and remove him when he is losing interest. It is a phase that some babies go through, and it passes. One of my babies bit everything – and everyone – for a while; it was embarrassing and I had to be careful, but he grew out of it. We carried on nursing.

So, while you can nurse a child with a mouth full of teeth and not get bitten, I also get calls from mothers asking for helpful suggestions because they are getting bitten, and they want to keep nursing. Sometimes babies will nip you if you offer the breast when they

need some other attention and you are fobbing them off with the thing that usually shuts them up!
Babies will chew on your fingers and their hands; they seem to prefer something soft to teeth on and sometimes it is a good idea to provide them with something – like a muslin nappy, to chew on.

I wonder if the reason our first teeth are called milk teeth is because they are present while we are receiving our mother's milk? Children are clearly designed to be breastfed for longer than our culture practises. The protective effect on milk teeth is obvious; my children had no visible plaque on their teeth until they stopped nursing. I nursed two of my children for several years, none have any fillings, and one of them is already an adult. Breastfeeding also influences the development of the shape of the jaw: it is more open in breastfed children, giving more space for adult teeth.

ILLNESS

Illness in the mother

Breastfeeding can continue through a mother's illness. Indeed, here is an important difference between breast and formula: continuing to breastfeed protects your baby from any infection you have by passing antibodies specific to that infection directly through the milk. The worst thing you could do would be to stop. So even if you feel awful, keep feeding and seek help. Mothers do worry that they will pass their illness on to the baby. Of course this is true, but it is quite deliberate. The baby catches the disease, is protected by the milk, and will be immune to it if it ever meets it again. This way our breastfed babies are stronger and less likely to be seriously ill.

One problem that occurs in a bottle feeding culture, is that we are so used to not taking food by mouth if we have a stomach bug, that we equate breastfeeding within this regime. It is true of formula feeding. However breastmilk is the perfect food to give a sick child, even when he can keep no other food down. It has the correct salt and sugar balance to prevent dehydration and it contains the antibodies to make the child well. It also keeps the iron necessary for bacterial growth available only to the baby, so by reverting to breastmilk alone the baby denies the infection the chance to develop. Usually the breastfed infant will ask to be constantly nursed until he feels better. Sometimes the only sign that your breastfed baby has been ill at all will be an increase in nursing, while other children (and adults) in the house may have been really unwell. This behaviour is not widely known to health professionals, so some misdiagnosis and suggestions of inappropriate weaning may be made.

While nursing my first child I had a stomach bug and lay limply in bed for several days. I hardly had the strength to lift my baby to feed her and could only drink water. She appeared unaffected.

If it is the mother who is affected by illness that requires drugs or hospitalization you may find it useful to telephone a breastfeeding counsellor to check the suitability of the drug you need while breastfeeding. Your doctor needs to know that you are feeding your baby. It is possible to find acceptable drugs to use while breastfeeding for all except thyroid and cancer treatments. It is also possible to take your breastfed baby with you into hospital while you need treatment. It may be suggested that you abruptly wean your baby. Mothers at this time feel that their baby needs them more than ever and are most reluctant to consider weaning. Sudden weaning at any time is not good for the mother either. You may need to explain how dependent your totally breastfed infant is on you and find a sympathetic medical professional. Some mothers have found the need to resort to private treatment so that they can have their baby with them. You will need a carer for the baby to bring him to you for feeding, and care for him while you are undergoing treatment.

Alternative therapies often answer the problem of finding safe treatments while breastfeeding and this is often a time when people start using them. I found homeopathic remedies particularly suitable and began using them when I had young children.
Please note however that because a remedy is alternative does not mean that it is safe for a baby. Check: for example some herbs are known to dry up milk and some essential oils are contraindicated during pregnancy.

Illness in the baby

Common infections in breastfed babies often pass unnoticed. Diseases with serious implications like whooping cough are significantly milder while breastfeeding, and not as distressing to the child. Any disease the mother has had as a child will mean that her baby will be quickly protected by her antibodies. If the mother has not had the disease herself her body will recognise it and produce antibodies for her baby in her breasts. These antibodies may never circulate in the mother's own bloodstream if she has not come into contact with the disease herself. The breast receives information about the disease from the baby and responds with the necessary antibody protection. Thus a crawling baby is protected by its mother's milk against diseases it may pick up as it automatically posts anything interesting looking into its mouth.

Breastmilk has special benefits for more complicated illness where the baby needs an operation or has a hereditary disease. It is digested easily, so it does not use much energy in the process. It protects from infection which means that the baby will recover more quickly from an operation or be less prone to infections which often beset children with conditions like Down's syndrome. Sadly many mothers are advised against breastfeeding babies with problems. This may be done to protect the parents from upset if their baby becomes very ill. In my experience however, parents wish to do the best for their children whatever the prognosis. Bonding with your baby is precious and the benefits human milk can bring these babies should not be underestimated.

Expressing milk

If your baby is unwell, especially if he is in Special Care after birth, you may need to express your milk. This is not necessarily as straightforward as it sounds, because breastfeeding a baby and pumping are not the same: the baby is much more efficient at getting the milk out. Women who know that they are producing lots of milk may only be able to express a little. Some women find it easier than others. If your baby is ill you will be determined, and that will help a lot.

I am going to give some basic guidelines here because mothers I speak to are unaware of how the system works, what stimulation is necessary and are often misinformed by staff on Special Care wards.

Additional information about using breastpumps or how to hand express is also available in "Bestfeeding : getting breastfeeding right for you" , Arms, Fisher and Renfrew.

It is important to express as often as you can – at least 1-3 hourly in the day and as often as you can at night. The times you express do not have to be at regular intervals. Do it when you can. I know that if your baby is in hospital and you are visiting as often as you can, you have to fit it in somewhere. The level of prolactin (milk producing hormone) is naturally higher at night so it is probably good to make use of it. I know that mothers separated from their babies often lie awake at night anyhow, so it is good to be able to do something useful for your baby. Don't worry if you produce an apparently tiny amount. A newborn tiny baby needs a teaspoon of colostrum (first milk produced by breasts during pregnancy and early postpartum, rich in antibodies) for a feed. If your baby is able to suck, offer the breast. If not, hold him close anyway and ask for tube or cup feeding, so that he won't prefer a bottle teat to your breast. If he does appear to prefer the teat it is because he has become used to the teat shape being already made for him and not because he does not 'like' you. Mothers can feel rejected if this happens.

Have your colostrum given first . It is given by syringe down the tube. Quantity is not important at this stage, but if you feel pressurized that your baby is not receiving enough fluid, you can ask for donated mother's milk to be given. Learning to feed can be tiring, but once the breast is letting down it is actually easier for a baby to feed from the breast than a bottle. Milk is squeezed out of the breast by muscles in the breast, so all the baby has to do is swallow (see Let-down). Any other sucking than on the breast, eg a dummy, discourages the baby from sucking well at the breast. It also prevents the breast from getting the stimulation it needs to produce milk.

Hand expression is a better mimic of a baby nursing than a pump, so it encourages the supply of milk better. Massage the breast first for several minutes, to warm it, increase blood flow and promote hormone release. This will also help you to relax and concentrate. Start by stroking the breast from the furthest points towards the nipple, all the way around. Lightly at first, especially if engorged, then with the palm of the hand. Express milk by closing thumb and fingers each side of the areola quite far up the breast from outside the areola and then close in towards the nipple. Work around the breast to drain all of the ducts. After a while you should get milk beginning to drip and then squirt out as the let down begins. When you have practised hand expression, you will find you get faster at it.

While pumping it can be helpful to have a photograph of your baby, listen to other babies crying, anything that will encourage hormone production to keep building a supply. Massage before pumping as for hand expression (see above). Pumping both breasts at a time is supposed to help hormone stimulation. The pump is not as effective as a baby at removing milk and does not give the feedback to the breast in the same way to increase production, so it can be difficult to keep producing a quantity of milk by pumping alone. However, if you are determined you will succeed. For the first few days however you have the advantage of the hormones from the birth, and you will produce milk whether you want it or not. If you can put your baby to the breast for only one feed a day to begin with it will help your supply. Cup feeding is a good substitute for, or progression from, tube feeding as the baby learns to use its mouth but does not learn a bottle sucking action.

A little cup (like a medicine cup) is used with a small amount of expressed milk in it. The cup is held to the baby's bottom lip, with the baby sitting upright, and tipped until the milk reaches his tongue. He will then gently sup it with his top lip. You have to be responsive to whether he wants more or not while tilting the cup. You do not pour it into his mouth, he takes what he wants as he is ready.

The mouth needs to be wider to take in the breast and it can be tricky once a baby has learned to take a bottle teat to get it to open up. It is possible though, so do not give up if this happens – find someone who can help you to reeducate your baby. It takes time and patience to do this, but the mothers who have say it is worth it and it gets easier.

Storing breastmilk

I am frequently asked about the storage of breastmilk. You can express into a container in the fridge for a day and keep the milk for the next day. It is best to give the milk as fresh as possible, although you can freeze it for up to 3 months. Some people freeze using ice cube trays so that you can defrost just what you need and not waste any.

Kangaroo Care

One method of care for small babies involves being tucked inside the mother's clothing next to her skin where they can feed on demand and stay warm. This successful method of care began in Columbia when there were not enough places in Neonatal units. Babies as small as two pounds are cared for in this way and the survival rate is very high in comparison with medical methods. It is occasionally practised in Britain. Even if the baby is not mature enough to nurse directly from the breast his presence encourages milk production and if he is not strong enough to nurse the mother can express milk directly into the baby's mouth by hand.
You don't need to have a sick baby to enjoy the closeness of carrying your baby, indeed, the feeling of nurturing you have is produced by prolactin – the same hormone that produces milk.

INFLUENCES

A study originally intended to ascertain whether working outside the home influenced a woman's decision to breastfeed discovered instead that the most influential factor upon her decision was the opinion of the father. 98% of women began breastfeeding if their partner supported this decision, only 27% when the father expressed no preference. This is a good example of the need for support among breastfeeding mothers. Even though bottle feeding involves a great deal more physical work, some women would rather face that than the uncertainty of making the decision to breastfeed alone. Women do sometimes think that if they bottle feed their menfolk will share the burden and take a turn at night feeding. Sadly this often turns out not to be the case, certainly after the first few weeks. Whether the father has work to return to or not, it is usually the mother who is left with the main task of childcare, irrespective of whether she returns to work herself.

Father's rôle

Those fathers who take a great interest in their partners' pregnancy and wish their baby to be breastfed often come to antenatal classes. I try to ensure that they attend the breastfeeding class because, quite understandably, they think that they need not be included. The father's rôle in the future health of his baby is to ensure that the baby is breastfed, so it is important that he knows about breastfeeding because he may have to defend it. I like to explain the mechanics of breastfeeding to both parents because then they stand a better chance of surviving the onslaught of different advice that they will probably receive, and remembering what they wanted to do when they set out. It is often the fathers who 'phone me now. That initial contact at the class is very useful. I am often asked if mothers should express milk and the fathers should give it to their baby in a bottle to make the job fair. My answer is this: babies have two parents with different rôles, the mother gives birth and produces milk and gets completely engrossed in her new status, especially the first time mother. The father is there to protect her in a vulnerable position, to provide for her and to fend off unwanted, unhelpful remarks that might damage her confidence at this time. He is a barrier between her and the outside world, which she needs when she has just given birth. It is a time when a woman – and both parents – are supposed to receive support from the family and wider community. The health of our children benefits us all. Babies love their mothers and need them to be there. They love their fathers in a different, but equally important, way. They need them to prove themselves to, to measure themselves up against and to be approved of by.

Some parents choose to take on different rôles: this is my view of the biological benefit of having two different parents serving different purposes.

They are not interchangeable. I also explain how these rôles are still relevant in these days of equality. Mothers often think that they should not ask for help. I suspect that this is to do with their professional lives, and the tendency for women to act in them like men. One of the most difficult things about new parenthood for professional women is that they are not in control, that they have to take on a rôle that they are not used to. They can find this threatening. To have a supportive partner with a sense of perspective and without a whole rush of hormones charging around his body as he has not just given birth, can be a real advantage.

Which of the jobs is he happy to do? What would the mother like him to do? The father may feel helpless when he cannot make everything alright to begin with – men in our society expect to be able to 'fix' things. What she may need is a back massage, supposed to help with the flow of milk when done between the shoulders, and heavenly in labour. The mother needs to be asked what would help and the father needs to know that he is being useful just by being willing.

Fathers can play a unique rôle in soothing babies. They are as loved and secure as the mother, but they are not confused about what is wrong with feeding and so uptight at the end of the day: the baby does not expect to be fed by his father. There is something very special about a man with his young baby and it can have a magical effect if the baby is fractious.

Another important rôle for the father, if the mother has had a Caesarean section or a lengthy delivery and is very tired, is to protect her from family and visitors until she is stronger. Breastfeeding can survive if the woman is dealing with the baby alone, but may be sacrificed if she feels pressure to entertain visitors or does not have enough privacy. You can work out a plan between you, about who is realistically helpful and who it would be best to keep away, or have very short visits from until later on. Some people are remarkably thick skinned at this time and the mother and baby can suffer. Be firm.

In dealing with those in authority, it is really useful for the mother to have the support of her partner. If a decision is seen as a joint decision she is much more likely to be respected when criticised.

It may seem to the fathers that their lives will never be private again, and of course they will never be quite the same, but the frantic time after the birth does pass. If the couple have been separated while the mother and baby have been in hospital, it may feel important to spend some time checking in with each other. The baby may seem to take priority too often. This happens with parents anxious to do everything properly. However, if you make the effort to keep communication open and enjoy each other's company, a baby can enrich your lives. There is a lovely description in a newsletter that I read recently written by a father explaining how he feels included into the special nursing relationship. As his wife nurses their baby, he arrives and the baby turns to smile at him and thus include him in their warm circle. If your relationship with your partner is strong, breastfeeding will not offer a threat to it.

Family and friends

How were you fed as a baby? It affects your confidence when it comes to breastfeeding yourself. What about your partner? The way his mother fed him will have a bearing on how supportive he is and how confident he is that you will succeed. Both your mother and his mother are powerful influences. They will have opinions about the introduction of solids, bottles of formula and whether you can cope. This last one is a challenge to deal with as concern can be catching, until you may wonder whether you really have taken on something impossible.

Make sure you have discussed what you feel happy with so that you can present a united front to your family and friends. You may find you have to deal with the expectations of everyone wanting to hold the baby perhaps, when you know he does not like it. I call this 'Pass the Baby' and I had trouble because I did not want to let other people hold my babies if they did not feel safe. I had quite a tussle with myself about whether it was OK to feel so protective that I did not want anyone to hold my new baby. Some people, especially grandmothers, may feel that they have a knack with babies, and think that if only you try what worked with hers everything will be alright. This belief can be undermining to your confidence when you are new to motherhood and not yet familiar with your own infant. I had to deal with a granny who was sure that a bottle would calm my troubled baby. Since she had bottle fed, it made sense to her to try this. However, it is not helpful to the new breastfeeding mother, and it does not solve any problems.

As you will probably be feeling tired in the early days, it can all seem a bit difficult to stick to breastfeeding when everyone may be thinking you are making life unnecessarily hard for yourself. This is the time when you and your partner need to hang onto what you had planned before and why it is so helpful to have read and discussed what you plan to do.

Having said this, it is possible to breastfeed without the support of partner and relatives and some women do this.

You may find that you can ask some relatives not to make unhelpful remarks. You may find that you have to see others less frequently until you are confident about what you are doing. It can be hard to defend breastfeeding at the beginning when you are learning what to do and the advantages are not obvious, even to you, and bottle feeding mothers appear to have their babies under strict control. Part of this is because the digestion of formula fat is incomplete and it sits in the baby's stomach making him feel still full when your breastfed baby will be asking for his next feed. It makes it seem as though your milk is not as satisfying, which is why some women succumb to giving supplementary feeds (see Differences between milks p.28).

If you are a single mother you may feel abandoned at this time. You may imagine every other new mother with a supportive partner while you struggle alone. There are advantages to being able follow your instincts and have no one to argue with, though people may worry about you coping alone. Bottle feeding is a lot more work and breastfeeding can be done automatically: if you are able to trust your body it is easier.

Breastfeeding organisations

The breastfeeding organisations exist to promote breastfeeding as the healthiest way to nurture our children. They may each have a slightly different angle on how to go about it, but the thing that they have in common is that they will support you in a way that is consistent with successful breastfeeding if you have a problem. They have a pool of experience that is invaluable, and access to considerable resources and expertise.

Many people try to offer a mother support by giving advice that is inconsistent with breastfeeding: giving supplements of formula instead of telling her how to increase her supply, for example, or suggesting nipple shields instead of getting the baby correctly latched onto the breast.

Another problem new mothers have to deal with in our fragmented society is isolation. Breastfeeding mothers may feel this more than most if they do not know other mothers who are breastfeeding. You can almost feel sometimes that people are blaming you for ostracizing yourself by choosing to breastfeed.

The breastfeeding groups can introduce you to other mothers who are breastfeeding. This is one of the best ways to keep motivated, and it is lovely if you can meet a mother who has nursed a previous child as well. I loved being with other women who were breastfeeding and it taught my children that it was normal.

The breastfeeding organizations are listed at the end of the book.

Society

Here in Britain the feeling that mothers often get is that they are expected to fail to breastfeed. It is revealed from the earliest stages when in pregnancy you are asked if you are going to 'try' to breastfeed. I found it hard to answer "Yes" firmly, even when I had already successfully breastfed. The accepted answer seems to be "Yes , if I can". It feels like a doubtful business.

When you have had a baby you become public property, everyone feels qualified and entitled to tell you how to look after your baby. Much as dog owners find people that they do not know will use the dog as an introduction and speak to them, strangers will walk up to you and make personal observations and ask searching questions, which even they might consider rude if you did not have a baby.

It takes a while to get over the shock and to learn how to handle this, mostly well- meaning, intrusiveness. I learned to keep several stock answers ready, which mostly did not answer the curious questioning, but did placate the inquirer so I could go on my way in peace. In answer to the question "Is she good?" (which means 'does she sleep all day and wake very seldom to be fed'), I used to say "I think she's lovely" or something equally evasive. I did not want to give them the chance to begin to tell me about how giving supplementary feeds would make her sleep. I wanted to breastfeed. She did wake frequently, she was not a happy baby and in the end I weakened and gave solids early. It made no difference at all, so I went back to solely breastfeeding.

It can feel like hard work to be breastfeeding in an unsupportive environment, if you are being questioned about what you are doing, you can begin to doubt yourself. A breastfeeding support group can become a haven for you to breastfeed without having to justify yourself. In British culture breastfeeding is not seen as natural, certainly not as normal. Bottle feeding and dummies are acceptable in public places whereas breastfeeding is not. If you begin to breastfeed someone may ask if you would like to go somewhere private, thus suggesting that what you are doing is seen as unacceptable.

Many women have reported to me that they were the only mother breastfeeding on the ward in the hospital where they had their baby. Several mothers have said it recently. It makes them feel like an object of curiosity, especially when members of staff come along and say "Oh, you're the one who's breastfeeding". It is difficult to keep your sense of purpose when you feel as if you have to perform. When it is the first time you have breastfed and you feel uncertain anyhow, the pressure can feel overwhelming. If you can, make contact with a breastfeeding support group before you have your baby. Then when you need some support you have already made contact.

In Norway breastfeeding has remained in favour. All babies are breastfed at birth and eighty per cent are still nursing at three months. It can be done in an industrialized country with supportive legislation for maternity leave and nursing breaks at work. There is actually a law in force in this country which allows a mother extra breaks to nurse her baby. Not many mothers are aware of it, however, and neither are many employers. Suitable payments for Child Benefit also need to be paid because at the moment a mother on a low income can get more if she leaves her child to go out to work. Although I have described how it is possible for a woman to go out to work and keep breastfeeding, many women would choose to look after their children if they felt they could afford to. It is easier to breastfeed if you are with your baby. In Norway it is also expected that your breastfeeding baby will come with you.

Breastfeeding in the media, especially on television, is rarely seen except in news or documentary coverage of communities during natural or political disaster – and far from home. I suspect that this leads many westerners to associate breastfeeding with poverty and perhaps starvation. Normal, everyday breastfeeding of bonny western babies is not shown. The power of the images presented in the media cannot be overestimated. They shape people's expectations and aspirations: breastfeeding is not something you can aspire to if you do not see it.

Health professionals and breastfeeding knowledge

I remember being told when I took my third child for his six week check up with a paediatrician that I had done well to breastfeed all my children. It was the first time any health worker had said such a thing and I was thrilled at being acknowledged. I also wondered why it so rarely happens?

The advice given to parents about breastfeeding is conflicting. They can become confused about what is the right thing to do when they are already feeling vulnerable. If you can find one person you trust and refer to them it helps. I suspect that much of midwife's and health visitor's knowledge comes from their personal experience. This may be useful if they breastfed successfully, although what worked for them may not for you. Unfortunately, many will not have fed successfully, which makes it harder for them to support you. A father recently expressed to me his disappointment with the fact that the midwife who gave the breastfeeding talk to the class that he attended with his wife had bottle fed her own children.

Breastfeeding support also involves spending time with each mother who needs assistance while establishing breastfeeding. Mothers often feel that their midwife does not have time to stay and assist them with breastfeeding. Since I estimate that it takes an hour to deal with a breastfeeding problem, this is probably correct.

My own lovely midwife fed her babies four hourly and told me that they slept for fourteen hours at night! This is obviously an extraordinary example of babies who fed seldom and a mother who could keep producing milk with very little stimulation. I could see she was tempted to suggest to me that I could persuade my son to do what her children had done, but he was my third and my children rarely fed less often than two hours or so. This midwife was very encouraging about breastfeeding and I heard had been criticized for spending too much time with mothers who needed help.

Professionals' training is improving and some midwives and health visitors have a special interest in breastfeeding and work hard to help mothers in their care. Extra training in areas of special interest is voluntary so their knowledge varies enormously. Doctors do not receive much training in the management of breastfeeding. This is only to be expected as it is not an illness and unless there is a problem we do not refer to them. They do however sometimes advise treatment inconsistent with successful breastfeeding management and are more familiar with bottle fed than breastfed infants. As we know, breastfeeding protects against illness so doctors see fewer breastfed babies. As a consequence of this children's wards in hospitals rarely have breastfed babies in them, and staff are not practised in how to deal with a breastfeeding couple if a breastfed baby should ever need to be admitted into hospital. Children in these wards are usually suffering from respiratory infections or gastroenteritis which breastmilk protects against.

The medical profession encouraged formula feeding earlier this century, as it was commonly believed that it was good for feeding to be regulated. A lot less was known about the special properties of breastmilk for human infants. The medical profession, however, is made up of people as much a product of the society they live in as the rest of us: but they suffer the extra burden of many of their patients wanting them to make decisions for them. This has gone on for so long that many are surprised by those parents who wish to make decisions about their children themselves. The medical profession also by its nature concentrates on illness, and mothers only come into contact with doctors when they have a problem. They are used to bodies going wrong so they may not trust them. Breastfeeding may then appear to be a lot more trouble than it is worth. It is difficult for women when someone they respect in other matters advises them in a way that they strongly disagree with about breastfeeding. This is a time when mothers may telephone me for moral support if they differ in opinion from their doctor.

Another potentially influential person I would like to mention is the nursing auxiliary. Staff on night duty in the hospital wards may not be trained midwives, or even nurses, and although they can be wonderfully supportive if they have successfully breastfed, it is the luck of the draw. If they have not, you may find yourself in the middle of the night feeling you have to justify your decision to breastfeed to someone who believes that the best solution to a crying baby is the most expedient one, ie giving a bottle of formula. They can have a brusque manner which is very upsetting to the mothers who have shared their experiences with me. They, like me, when I had my first baby had no idea that these women were not trained professionals, and were bewildered by the nature of the treatment they received from them.

The biggest disservice that the medical profession has done to the public is to suggest that there is no difference between breastmilk and formula, which is essentially what happens if you think it merely a matter of practical choice of feeding method. I believe parents need to be aware that in this matter the scales are tipped heavily in one direction and that those parents who wish their babies to be breastfed deserve all the support and information that we can give.

ADVANTAGES TO THE MOTHER OF BREASTFEEDING

So far I have mostly talked about the advantages of breastfeeding for the baby. Surprisingly perhaps, this is one of those parenting tasks where the best thing for the baby can also be the easiest for the mother.

Convenience

Breast milk is available anytime, anywhere, with no extra work on the part of the mother. From a lengthy traffic jam on a motorway to an isolated mountain, anywhere you go with your baby the food is always available, and you need take nothing with you. Travelling by aeroplane is eased by nursing your baby on take off and landing, holiday plans need no special equipment. In a power cut or water shortage you can still feed your baby. You do not need to get up in the night to feed your baby, you can feed him with your eyes shut and in your sleep. Breastfed children often do not get as ill and do not get as distressed when they do.

The soothing effect of nursing calms a tired child, a teething infant, a bumped toddler and a frightened baby. My friend mentioned nursing her seven month old during a thunder storm; he was terrified but nursing calmed him immediately.

If your child needs medical treatment that is painful, nursing can offer pain relief and security. It is sometimes the only thing you can do in a difficult situation, it is such a relief to be able to. I remember my realization as I talked to a bottle feeding mother about her child's illness. The baby had sickness and diarrhoea, and the mother could give her nothing. I was horrified as I thought of the distress to me as well as to my children if I could not nurse them when they were ill. Breastmilk is the perfect food for a sick child, even when they can eat nothing else.

The baby does not equate the breast with getting fed, only with feeling better. So whatever their reason for feeling in need, the breast is their source of comfort. Happily, the design of the system is such that whatever the baby requests from the breast, the baby will be correctly nourished.

A breastfed baby may pass a motion every feed or once a week – I think it can be called a convenience if it is once a week, but you get what you get. There is nothing you can do about it. See Expectations p.38.

Another convenience for the mother that many people do not realize is that a woman usually does not menstruate while she is fully breastfeeding, certainly for the first few months, sometimes for many months. It must be difficult to be dealing with having periods when you have a new baby to look after.

Health

There are specific health benefits to nursing mothers, research has demonstrated fewer urinary tract infections, reduced cancer of the breast and ovaries, and fewer hip fractures in the elderly. While the mother's body is involved in protecting the infant from infection it also protects her own.

The absence of periods contributes to a mother's health, when she does not want to be conceiving again as she has a young baby. Fertility may return before periods however, the period of breastfeeding merely delays further conception until the infant is feeding less frequently. It has been estimated that by full, long-term breastfeeding alone the contraceptive effect of breastfeeding would mean that the average woman would have five or six children.

Satisfaction

The satisfaction of nursing your baby is huge, it is an enormous sense of achievement to know that you have provided the perfect food for your growing child. The process itself is really enjoyable. You inevitably talk to your baby, hold his hands and toes and generally enjoy the opportunity to interact. The physical sensations during breastfeeding are experienced by some mothers as pleasurable too. It makes sense to me that something so important to the welfare of our children should be enjoyable.

If a mother has satisfactorily breastfed one child she will do it again. At a breastfeeding meeting I attended once a mother said: "No one told me it would be wonderful!".

Self image

Breastfeeding uses the stores of fat laid down for the purpose. It also gives a sense of value to you about your body, because you are responsible for nourishing your baby.

Some women feel guilty about the fact that they avoid a lot of extra work by breastfeeding. They call themselves 'lazy' mothers. It seems to me to be an intelligent thing to nurse your baby, which is definitely better for him, and to have energy left to enjoy him. Looking after your first baby particularly, is challenging enough without the extra work of preparing formula feeds. One counsellor expressed to me that she gets the impression that a woman is considered a better mother if she gets up in the night, warms bottles and paces the floor to settle her baby rather than snuggling up to nurse her baby in the comfort of her bed. I can think of no advantage to the baby of the mother being a martyr.

I feel the same way about women forcing themselves to continue to breastfeed or whatever they think they ought to do to be the 'perfect' parent. Resentment is the worst thing you can offer your child. Do whatever is the most joyful option you have. Once you stop forcing yourself, you might even find that you can enjoy doing whatever you felt was such hard work when it was a duty. Finding support while you are breastfeeding can change your feeling about it entirely, you do not need to plough on alone. Making friends who are also breastfeeding is supportive and satisfying and helps your child.

Another advantage, rarely mentioned, is the fact that breastfed babies' nappies don't smell awful. Breastmilk is almost entirely digested and until your baby moves onto mixed feeding you have the advantage of not being aesthetically assaulted every time you change a nappy.

WHAT TO DO IF YOU HAVE PROBLEMS

I have endeavoured to cover some common problems encountered by breastfeeding couples here, it is not intended to be comprehensive. The message I would like to convey is that 'where there is a will there is a way' with breastfeeding. It is almost always possible to overcome problems and temporary hiccups that may seem impassable at the time, but with the right knowledge and support will leave you glad that you did not give up, and continuing to enjoy the special breastfeeding relationship you have with your baby.

Inverted nipples

If your nipples point in when you stand naked in a cold bathroom then they are called inverted. With a willing baby this may make no difference to your ability to breastfeed. A much bigger portion of the breast is taken into the baby's mouth during breastfeeding than just the nipple. So that once the baby is latched on, the nipple is pulled out and functions normally. Breasts do change during pregnancy, and sometimes the nipples visibly alter during this time. Some women have one nipple that is inverted, and once the baby has learned to latch onto the standard one it has no trouble with the inverted one. When the baby comes off the breast you can see the inverted nipple looking pointed for a while afterwards.

Sometimes it takes longer to latch a baby on when both nipples are inverted, but it is perfectly possible. Remember that many babies take a while to learn how to latch on, whatever shape their mothers' breasts are. People come in all shapes and sizes and if a body type really did not work it would have died out.

Some women try specific exercises during pregnancy; there are some gadgets purported to change inverted nipples. Having met some women who have fed their babies successfully with inverted nipples, I suspect that it is more a matter of patience in allowing the baby to learn to latch on. An extensive research into treatment during pregnancy for flat or inverted nipples concluded that there was no benefit from wearing breast shells or doing nipple stretching exercises. It is certainly not true that having inverted nipples means that you cannot breastfeed, as used to be thought the case. Mothers used to have their breasts inspected during pregnancy and were told whether their nipples were suitable for breastfeeding or not. This did nothing to boost their confidence when they may already have been feeling uncertain, and shows the lack of trust that is generally felt about the human body.

Sore nipples

A common problem with early breastfeeding is soreness. There are several reasons for this:

1) Unfamiliarity. Women in our culture are not used to any sensation on their breasts as they usually wear a bra that allows no movement and layers of clothes to keep warm. It takes a while to get used to nursing a baby on skin that is not usually exposed even to the rubbing of clothes, and certainly not to the elements, as our hands and faces are. Even the normal pinching sensation of the baby latching on feels strange to begin with.

2) Incorrect positioning. Breastfeeding should not hurt once the baby is latched on and is suckling correctly. Even if the skin is already damaged, and then the correct position is adopted, it will stop hurting after the initial latch on. Take him off the breast if it is hurting (put your little finger into the corner of his mouth to break the suction), wait until he turns with his mouth wide open, pull him quickly onto the breast while his mouth is as wide as he will open it. You can also try putting more breast into the baby's mouth – while he is on the breast – by posting it in from

underneath. If you have no joy finding a health professional able to help you to latch satisfactorily you may 'phone a breastfeeding counsellor.

3) Ignoring the pain. Women ignore the warning signs and continue to nurse and allow the baby to damage the breast. Often this is because they are so afraid that he will not latch on again that they continue incorrectly because at least he is nursing. Professional knowledge is thin on the ground. Women are sometimes advised that the baby is correctly latched on when the pain the mother is feeling clearly states that he is not. The mother is not in a position to argue at a time like this: she does not know that it is not supposed to hurt.

4) Engorgement. A very full breast is difficult for a baby to draw into his mouth to begin to nurse. He will apply as much suction as is necessary – and sometimes it is a lot. The breast is more easily bruised when overfull. It can help to express a little milk and have a bath. It is a situation best avoided if you can. See Engorgement p.133.

5) Baby's mouth size. To start off with the breast is bigger than the baby's head and he may have trouble getting all the breast he needs into his little

mouth. It may take several tries each feed to get latched on, so that he has enough breast in his mouth to milk the breast effectively. The baby grows quickly and the breast diminishes in size quite naturally as the balance of supply and demand emerges.

Many women have a temporary soreness while the breast gets used to the baby suckling. I guess that the skin is renewed several times a day as the baby nurses. What needs to happen is that you are renewing the skin slightly faster than the baby is wearing it off. The same is true of any area of the body that does physical work – palms of hands, lips etc. – and we only notice a problem if the replacement time gets out of synchronization with the wear and tear. I liken it to wearing a new pair of shoes and getting blisters if you keep wearing them when you are getting sore heels. There are certain measures that you can take to help, but do not let them stop you from getting the positioning right. This is fundamental to preventing further problems.

Remedies for soreness:
(i)   Correct positioning
(ii)   Fresh air
(iii)   Calendula cream (not lanolin based)

(iv)   Light

(v)   Vitamin E

(vi)   Avoid iron tablets

(vii)   Breastmilk

(viii)   Alternative feeding position

(i) I have covered correct positioning. See: Latching on p.18, as well as comments above.

(ii) Fresh air seems to help skin damage to heal, either leave off bra and wear loose clothing or tea strainers in the bra with the handles cut off. Avoid breast pads as they can perpetuate soreness.

(iii) Calendula cream is sold as a cut cream, not specifically for breastfeeding (sometimes sold as Hypercal, you will find it in Health Food shops and Boots homeopathic range). I have found it speeds up the healing process remarkably, which is really useful when you know your baby is going to want to feed again shortly. Avoid the lanolin based one; some women are allergic to it and that makes their problem worse, it is also sticky whereas the non-lanolin based one is quickly absorbed. You only need to put a trace on.

(iv) Sunlight and daylight are ideal, even through

glass. If you are in the middle of winter as you read this you can use artificial light. You only need a short exposure to really help the healing process: a minute or less at eighteen inches from a bare light bulb. Be careful not to over expose already delicate skin.

(v) Vitamin E is the vitamin we use to keep our skin flexible and reduce inflammation, it is also used in a number of other important body functions. Cold pressed oil is the easiest way to get it, wheat germ and safflower are particularly rich. You can eat it and put it onto the skin. See Diet p.79.

(vii) Excess iron destroys vitamin E and can lead to soreness. Iron is easily obtained in the diet and if you need to build your reserves up you can eat molasses, dried apricots, nuts – particularly almonds, watercress, spinach and wholemeal bread. Iron absorption depends on eating enough vitamin C.

(vii) Breastmilk allowed to dry on the skin is soothing and helps it to heal.

(viii) Alternative feeding positions offer some respite to the damaged area as the baby latches on. You can try putting his body under your arm, feeding while lying down (see description of sleeping with a baby p.56), or putting him on your tummy – in the bath is nice. These positions will vary the place under stress and allow it to heal, even though the baby will probably still be nursing frequently. Feeding from the least sore side first will mean that he is not as hungry and less likely to damage the sore side further.

Some women find honey beneficial, others find that the nipple needs to be kept moist as drying makes the skin crack. You will have to try these suggestions to see which work for you.

Find someone who is breastfeeding happily and ask if you can look at the position of their baby on the breast. There are some helpful pictures in books and on video that show correct positioning well (see "Bestfeeding: getting breastfeeding right for you" and the Royal College of Midwives video "Successful Breastfeeding"). There are also some that show incorrect positioning so do not assume that all the photographers know about breastfeeding.

Soreness can be a misnomer: the pain of feeding with damaged nipples is excruciating and mothers frequently end up in tears over it, worried that the baby will starve if they stop to put things right, and about their disappointment if they give up.

Cracked nipples

Cracked nipples are a further development from soreness and the treatment is as above for sore nipples. The nipples may bleed and parents worry if their baby is swallowing some blood. This is not harmful to the baby but obviously the situation needs to be attended to as soon as possible. Sometimes it can help to express milk for a day because it hurts too much for the mother to be able to put the baby to the breast. Pumps are available for hire from the breastfeeding organizations, or your health visitor may be able to get hold of one for you. (Try the 'phone book for local groups or the national addresses.)

Nipple Shields

Nipple shields are often suggested to mothers as a method for getting a baby to take the breast. Unfortunately they can cause more problems than they alleviate. Latching on is best achieved with patience and confidence that the baby will eventually take the breast – especially if not given anything else to suck on in the meantime. Nipple shields appear to give a quick solution to the problem of a baby who is taking time to learn to suckle. Breastfeeding is not necessarily a speedy business, especially in the first few days. Sometimes they are offered if a woman is experiencing soreness, which would probably be alleviated by correct positioning.

The disadvantages of nipple shields are:
1) That babies will later refuse to feed without them
2) That they restrict the flow of milk to the baby and
3) That they prevent full stimulation of the breast to produce more milk.

They are therefore not advised long term. The problem parents contact me about is trying to get the baby to latch onto the breast without them. Some ingenious solutions to this problem have been found, from putting sterilizing solution onto the breast so it smells familiar to the baby, to cutting a millimetre a day off the end of the shield until there is just a ring left and the baby is fully fixed to the breast. I have even had a call from a mother who fully breastfed each of her four children with a nipple shield for every feed. That seems to rather defeat the idea that breastfeeding can be more convenient, but I admired her perseverance.

Nipple shields are occasionally useful when cracked nipples are too painful to nurse from for a day. Obviously it would be better not to get so damaged in the first place.

Engorgement

This painful overfilling of the breasts with fluid and extra blood supply as well as milk, is so common about the third day after birth that many people think of it as normal. However it is preventable by nursing your baby soon after birth and frequently during the early days. If you are having your first baby you may not know about avoiding it. If you are having a subsequent baby you will realize that letting your baby sleep is not as pressing a need as making sure that breastfeeding gets off to a good start. The temptation to wrap babies up in an already overheated environment I suspect makes them sleepier, so unwrapping may make them more alert to feed. You can make sure that yours is warm enough by holding him in your arms with relatively few clothes on. Your body heat is the ideal temperature and your movements may alert him to feed more. Frequent short feeds are best for the baby and you at this stage.

If you already have engorgement, it is natural to feel upset and rather helpless. You have all this milk but you can't seem to get the baby to drink: it is really frustrating. You can express some milk to give the baby a chance to grasp the nipple. Hand expression all around the breast may be gentler: the swollen breast is vulnerable to bruising. The homeopathic remedy for bruising, Arnica, is useful at this time as is Calendula for soreness. Baths and showers can help by allowing some milk to leak because of the warmth; try expressing in the bath. Savoy cabbage leaves can also be used to soothe the breast (tucked into the bra) or cold flannels. A bath is also a wonderful opportunity for you to feed your baby in a new, relaxing environment. It works with all sorts of problems, and it is lovely anyway. Babies will often latch on in the bath who are otherwise reluctant and then go on to feed more happily.

Blocked duct

If you find that one part of a breast is not emptying, it feels hard and may look red, then one of the ducts is blocked. The breast is made up of sections, each leading to one of the eleven or so ducts, to the nipple. If you bruise the breast in some way it leads to a swelling and may cause an obstruction of one or more ducts. Keep feeding and massage the breast. This may be all you need to do to clear a blocked duct. Also see below: Mastitis, for what I have discovered works to clear up breast inflammation.

You may feel upset and imagine that you will have to stop feeding. Lots of women have blocked ducts and continue to nurse successfully. It is not a good time to stop, even if you had planned to begin weaning.

If you can discover what caused the blockage in the first place you can prevent it recurring. Some causes are:
• Ill fitting bra, digging in, often under the arm
• Badly designed bra, with part of the cup lowering to feed and the other part cutting across the duct as the

milk lets down
• Sleeping awkwardly on the breast for too long
• Toddler jumping enthusiastically on your lap and bumping the breast
• Knocking the breast during everyday movement

The lactating breast is vulnerable to bruising, which is why it is useful that the breasts are protectively situated between our arms on our chests. I have noticed that bruising on the breast is not the characteristic blue colour that you get on muscular areas, it goes red instead and I think that's why we don't always realize that we have bruised a breast. If there is any swelling then the larger fat molecules in the milk may not be able to flow through the duct and so it becomes blocked. If you keep feeding the baby and gently massaging from the outside of the breast along the ducts to the nipple the force of the let down will clear the blockage.

Mastitis

Mastitis is the technical word for inflammation of the breast. It can include infection.
The symptoms are the same as for a blocked duct but

you may feel unwell – as if you have 'flu; high temperature, weak, tired. The breast is red and the skin often shiny. The pain can be relieved by feeding the baby, there is no danger to the baby from drinking the milk because the infection is not present in the ducts. The inflammation may not be due to an infectious invasion. If you follow the suggestions below, you may avoid the need for antibiotic treatment, which can make your baby unwell and lead to other problems for you. I say this because the 'flu-like symptoms can be caused by the mother's body's reaction to her own milk escaping into her bloodstream and being recognized by her immune system as foreign protein. If the tiny milk sacs become over filled some may burst and some milk then mixes with her blood which is not normally the case. The two systems are designed to work separately. So her body treats the milk protein as an infectious invasion and raises her temperature to remove it. It is possible that the mother has an infection, but I have found that these remedies allow the body to heal itself. If it persists however and you feel ill for more than forty eight hours I would suggest that you seek medical attention. Sometimes the mastitis is due to an infection from elsewhere and requires antibiotic treatment. This can be discovered by taking a sample of the milk for laboratory examination. Make sure your doctor knows that you are breastfeeding if he prescribes drugs for you.

My methods for unblocking ducts and preventing infection developing:

KEEP BREASTFEEDING
Massage the breast (see below)
Take Arnica (for bruising) cream to massage into the breast and available in homeopathic tablets
Take vitamin E (reduces inflammation)
and Vitamin C (prevents infection)
Rest if you feel fatigue
Fenugreek tea, bitter but effective

Breast massage is done with the heel of the hand from the perimeter of the breast towards the nipple all the way around. If the breast is really tender, start very lightly and increase pressure as the breast gets used to it. Following the line of the ducts helps the milk to flow through the blocked area. Massaging with arnica cream reduces swelling quickly.

Abscess

If mastitis is not correctly treated – especially if the mother is advised to stop breastfeeding – an abscess can develop that needs surgical treatment. It is possible to keep nursing, sometimes you need to express and dispose of milk from the affected breast. But often you can keep nursing as the baby is protected against any infection that might get into the milk by your antibodies. If the wound from the incision to drain the abscess is not too close to the nipple you may be able to keep nursing all the time from the affected breast. More information than I want to cover here about these conditions is available from breastfeeding counsellors and books like Breast is Best or Bestfeeding.

Crying

Crying shows that a baby is in great distress. Usually before a baby cries he has endeavoured to express what he needs in other ways; by muttering or slurping on his hand hopefully, for example. It is therefore often possible to avoid the need for your baby to cry. I am saddened by the notion that babies automatically cry. I remember hearing the sound effects department of the

BBC being described on the radio some years ago. The universally accepted indication that a baby was present in a radio play was the sound of it crying. Is it so ordinary for us to leave our babies in distress that we consider it acceptable? Babies make lots of other delightful noises that could be used instead.

By saying all this I am suggesting that if your baby is crying incessantly and you are worried, then there may very well be something wrong with him. The problem sometimes is to get someone to understand that you do not consider it normal behaviour in your baby. Mothers are usually pretty good at knowing if there is something wrong with their child.

I am also saying that it is fine to give your child what he needs when he asks quietly. You are not doing him any harm by giving him what he needs before he yells. That just means he loses faith in you. It is fortunately no longer in fashion to ignore babies' cries for hours on end because it was not time for them to be fed. The myth that you can harm your baby by giving him what he needs still persists in some minds though. Sometimes our own. Mothers do 'phone me to ask if it is OK to give the baby everything he wants sometimes. My answer is that with a young baby , if you give him everything he needs, then he will become a trusting and independent child. I can say that now. I waited until my eldest was ten before I dared to admit that what I had believed in might have worked.

Different types of cry mean different things and you soon learn what your baby needs by his cry. Some babies have a need to be held a lot, a baby carrier is useful if you have a child who is afraid when left. Some babies just do cry when they are tired and dropping off to sleep. Others cry when frightened or have tummy ache, some hardly cry at all. I found that if I did not know what was wrong, the way to deal with it was to hold the child while she cried because then she knew I was there. Sometimes it was very hard because I had a child that cried for many hours. I was advised to put her in her pram at the bottom of the garden so I could not hear her. But I did not want to not hear her. I did not want her to be so upset. I was at my wit's end with this baby that screamed for hours without stopping. In the end I took her to all the clinics to try to find help before I damaged her in my frustration – yes, a baby's cry is not supposed to be ignored – I had a doctor who said 'You didn't expect to have a baby that didn't cry did you?'. None of the people I spoke to had any answers, she eventually grew out of it but I did not discover what her problem had been for another two babies...

Colic

This word is used to describe a collection of symptoms of a baby in distress. It includes crying bouts, screaming, drawing up of the knees and a desperation which is very upsetting to be around. It inevitably results in a lack of feeding and sleep – for everyone. Some babies cry miserably when put down and lonely but quieten down when held. A baby with colic carries on screaming as if someone were sticking pins into it. I remember checking to make sure the nappy pin was not sticking into her. Later, much later, I discovered that she was allergic to me drinking cow's milk. It obviously gave her terrible stomach pains which she could not tell me about because she was too young to talk. Some colic may be caused by food in the mother's diet. If it is a 'one off', it may be something unusual, that you do not eat every day. One of my babies was upset if I ate strawberries or melon. In this case it is fairly easy to identify and not to eat, particularly in large quantities, while nursing. If your baby screams for periods each day, it may be due to something you eat every day. Sometimes you can pinpoint it by the time they are distressed. Reactions usually take twelve hours. However, sometimes they are much faster.

If your child also has a runny nose, cough, is often sick or has rashes he may well be allergic. These symptoms are typical of cow's milk allergy, but may also be due to egg or nuts. Some babies are upset by large quantities of coffee, tea, cola or other stimulants.

I suggest that a mother only cuts a food out of her diet if she is fairly sure it is causing a problem. Generally it is best to eat a moderate amount of a wide variety of foods.

Above all, get support, and keep asking until you find out what is wrong. Babies are not supposed to scream on and on, and you are not a bad mother if you cannot put up with it. As I said before, a baby's cry is not supposed to be pleasant, and if you cannot help your baby you feel utterly dejected and helpless.

There are medical conditions that cause colic symptoms, like abnormalities or obstructions of the gut, so it is worth getting him checked by a doctor if you believe something is wrong.

Thrush

Whether or not you are prone to thrush, you may find that you have it at some point while breastfeeding. Thrush is a fungal infection that thrives on moist areas of the body when the acid balance has been altered. It only affects the nipples during the period of breastfeeding because the nipples are then regularly moist. The signs are usually itching and soreness of the nipples – sometimes accompanied by pain through the breast – and following feeding, after a period of trouble free breastfeeding . The baby may have a red mouth, and a white substance inside his cheeks. Do not confuse this with the white stain on his tongue from the milk after he has fed. He may have no symptoms at all. Thrush is not serious, and breastfeeding need not be affected, even though it may take several weeks to clear it up.

You both need to be treated. In mild cases there is a topical remedy that you can use to put on your nipples and in your baby's mouth. Use a solution of 1 teaspoon of bicarbonate of soda in a cup of water on a cotton wool swab to wipe the baby's mouth after each feed. Also bathe your nipples after nursing with a solution of 1 tablespoon of vinegar to a cup of water.

If there is no improvement after a few days, consult your doctor. You may find some confusion in doctors who are only used to seeing thrush in formula fed infants. The symptoms are not quite the same. You may need to take a systemic treatment if the thrush has invaded the ducts.

You can help your body to withstand thrush by avoiding white sugar and eating some live yoghurt (there are alternative yoghurts if you are sensitive to cow's milk).

Tongue tie

I am mentioning this here, because although relatively uncommon, it seems difficult to identify and get treatment.

The baby with tongue tie cannot effectively breastfeed because the tongue needs to be well extended to grasp the breast and work the milk out. In this condition the tongue is too closely linked to the bottom of the mouth by the frenulum (thin membrane under the tongue), which runs to the end of the tongue instead of finishing about half way along and enabling the baby to stick out its tongue. The tongue appears heart-shaped when extended and the baby makes clicking sounds as it sucks because it cannot make an airtight seal or get far enough onto the breast. The tongue needs to be able to extend far enough to go out over its bottom lip. The mother is also usually in considerable pain as the baby sucks hard without being able to get properly onto the breast.

Parents find it difficult to get this treated. It is a simple procedure to cut part of the frenulum, but no longer automatically done as it does not interfere with bottle feeding. I understand that it is usually treated to enable proper speech to develop at about eighteen months, though I would have said that it would be advisable for that reason much sooner as some babies experiment with recognizable language from about seven months.

I understand that in babies with tongue tie midwives used to cut the frenulum freeing it and making breastfeeding possible straightaway. I think the answer if you have this problem is to keep asking until you find a doctor or paediatrician who is sympathetic to breastfeeding.

Cleft lip and palate

After the initial shock and disappointment of discovering that you do not have the perfect baby that you imagined, try to remember that the corrective surgery for this condition is excellent – usually the repair is unnoticeable later – and that your baby needs your milk to ensure that he recovers as quickly as possible.

It is possible to breastfeed a baby with a cleft lip;and there are devices available to seal off a cleft palate to enable the baby to breastfeed. Others use their finger to fill the gap so that the baby can maintain suction. This may only need to be done for a short while if the baby is due to have an operation, which may be done only days after the birth. Feeding needs to be done upright, slowly, to give the baby a time to swallow. Some mothers find that they can express into the baby's mouth. Others pump their milk and give it by spoon or bottle with a special teat. These conditions are described in Breast is Best and the larger breastfeeding manuals – the La Leche League have a comprehensive one. The breastfeeding organizations will be able to help you. See Expressing milk p93.

SPECIAL CIRCUMSTANCES

Caesarean section

While Caesarean sections have become commonplace, they are nevertheless a major operation, and need to be recognized as such. Many women express to me the unexpected nature of the pain and immobility they feel after a Caesarean. Breastfeeding is more difficult when you can hardly move and your body needs to heal. Your milk may take up to a week to come in – that is for the mature milk to flow – before this you will be able to feed your baby colostrum. The hormones necessary for milk production are usually triggered by labour, so your body will take longer to adjust if you did not go into labour at all. Your milk will be stimulated by the baby sucking.

Many mothers who have had Caesareans end up having not begun to breastfeed as they planned, and starting later. This is possible, and with determination you will succeed. It is important to have help. One antenatal teacher I know visited one of the members of her class in hospital. She found that the mother had been left with a tray of food at the end of the bed and her baby in a cot, she could reach neither and was upset. The teacher was distressed to find a mother left in this state. Sadly, the staff are not numerous enough to cover the wards effectively, and when mothers receive help it is not always in the way that they need.

If you have had a Caesarean section, you may find it more comfortable to feed your baby lying down on your side. Some mothers put a pillow on their lap to lift the baby and keep it away from their stitches. Your partner may put the baby to your breast if you are unable to soon after birth.

Twins and more

It is perfectly possible to feed a baby from one breast only, and therefore to feed twins. Triplets are harder, you can only ever feed two at a time, but quite possible. With the amount of work looking after multiple babies, breastfeeding cuts out one huge chore. I read Di McDonald's account of breastfeeding triplets when I was expecting my third baby and it made me feel much better about the prospect of three children to look after. It is indeed a useful account because there are still women being told that it is not possible to feed twins. Try Di McDonald "More than One".

An Australian study demonstrated how mothers of twins were capable of producing several pints of milk a day to feed their breastfed twins solely for the first six months or so.

Since many twins are smaller than average, and a fair number premature, you may have babies in Special Care and be expressing for a while (see Expressing p.93). Putting your babies to the breast or even holding them close to you if they are not ready to nurse can stimulate your supply and let down reflex.

If you are expecting twins TAMBA (formerly the Twins Club) may be able to put you in touch with a local mother who has breastfed her twins. The breastfeeding organisations (see Useful addresses) will also be able to support you.

Working and Breastfeeding

Many people assume that a woman cannot continue to breastfeed after she returns to work.

Contrary to popular belief, studies have shown that a greater number of women continue to breastfeed when they return to work than those who do not. This may be related to the type of women who have a job to which they plan to return and therefore also be the type of women who might be expected to continue breastfeeding. However it shows that women are finding the value of breastfeeding for themselves, wanting to continue and discovering means to do so.

It is quite possible to continue exclusively breastfeeding when you return full-time, by expressing milk during the day, to be given to your baby the following day. Part-time work can mean that you feed before and after work, maybe not needing to express at all. Returning two full days means that you may express on the other days for those two, and express at work to avoid discomfort or to save the milk for work days. There are many approaches, all you need to know at the outset is that it can be done, then work out a scheme that will work for you. Try "The Breastfeeding Guide for the Working Woman". This is one of several books that contains information about storage of breastmilk.

Expressing milk is not necessarily straightforward. It may take practice. The availability of breast pumps suggests to people that it is automatic to be able to express all the milk you need to. The pump is not as efficient as the baby. When you are out at work the other feeds of the day taken directly from the breast by the baby help to maintain supply by contact with the breast. Some women find that what works better for them is if the baby is brought to them during the day to be fed or if they have a work-place nursery.

The women I speak to usually plan to return when their baby is between four and six months old. They sometimes worry a great deal about how the baby will be fed, thinking that he will have to get used to bottles of formula. They sometimes try to give bottles to their baby at about 2 months to get them used to it, and end up with a frantic and furious baby, who wonders what their breastfeeding mother is playing at. They then telephone me in desperation.

If you want your baby to have bottles, try getting someone else to do it. If you would prefer not to give your baby bottles, then there are other ways to give drinks. Some babies are given formula while their mothers are out at work during the day, and breastfed when with their mothers. Your baby does not need to have formula at all, if this is what you would prefer. This is the sort of age when some babies will happily take water in a beaker with a spouted lid, they may also be willing to eat some food. Let the baby guide you. Panicking about what might happen, or trying to predict what your baby will be ready for in 3 months time is useless. A few weeks before you may have some idea about whether your baby is likely to be solely breastfed still, and if you are going back to work some distance away, then you need to work out a plan for expression and storage. Remember though, babies can mature in big leaps, and may be ready for something you had not imagined only a few weeks previously.

You will have to make childcare workers aware that you want your child to have breast milk because it is still fairly unusual to have a breastfed baby in a nursery. Breastfed babies continue to nurse from their mothers when they are available, in the morning and evening, and at night. This is useful to keep up your supply. The baby may well want more feeds at those times than before you returned to work, and sometimes will begin to wake again at night, if he had stopped. This is all quite normal, and a good reason for being able to sleep while nursing.

One mother I spoke to was worried because her baby

would not take anything apart from breast milk from her before she returned to work. He refused everything at first while she was away during the day. Then after a few weeks he began to eat lunch, but would only have breast milk from his mother
to drink. She reported that he seemed perfectly well. My friend returned to work while still nursing her one year old. He liked to nurse as soon as she got home and she enjoyed the chance to sit with him and unwind.

Obligatory breastfeeding breaks are on statute in this country. If women make use of them, it will become easier for those who follow to keep breastfeeding.

Adoption

Some women choose to breastfeed their adopted babies. It takes preparation: expressing several times a day for some weeks before your baby arrives. It is also uncertain because you do not know if your adopted baby will take to the breast, but the fact that some women have done it shows that it can be done. Since the production of breastmilk relies on stimulation it is possible to produce milk without having recently had a baby. Perseverance is required, from the expression of milk with no baby there at all at first, to teaching the baby to breastfeed – the time and success rate involved will vary depending on how old the baby is and how determined you are! Mothers who have breastfed their own children previously may find they are able to produce enough milk to breastfeed exclusively. Those who have never had a baby may find that they can produce a proportion of their adoptive baby's necessary milk. While building your supply, once you have the baby nursing from you, a nursing supplementer may be useful. A tube attached to the breast next to the nipple delivers milk from a bottle hung by a cord around the mother's neck. This enables the baby to stimulate the breast while getting something to eat straightaway.

The relationship created by breastfeeding is clearly a huge motivation in a mother who is adopting and planning to breastfeed, as well as the superior nutrition. It helps to feel that you have done something very personal and special for your adoptive child. The bond it creates is a powerful one. Once a baby is nursing from you, you need the baby in the same way as it needs you. People are often surprised that it is possible to feed a baby that is not your own. This has been done through the ages and is another survival mechanism where a baby can be taken care of if its own mother dies. In some cultures it is quite acceptable for a woman to feed another's baby or toddler if she happens to be more available. In this country sometimes sisters will feed each others' children when they babysit for example. Wet nursing was common when noble women delegated feeding their children – this may have been as much so that they could have more children quickly as to save them the trouble of nursing their own. In some cultures the grandmothers feed the babies so that the mothers can return to work, because a younger woman can earn more.

Support for special breastfeeding situations is available from the breastfeeding organisations.

Relactation

Some women wish to return to breastfeeding having stopped for some time.

The breasts need to be stimulated to begin to produce milk again. If your baby only stopped nursing very recently and is willing to suckle you will find your milk returning in a matter of days. Indeed it takes many months for the breasts to stop making milk completely when you have been breastfeeding for a long time. The return to full lactation will take longer but if the baby is allowed free access to the breast this may only be a week or two (the Nursing supplementer may be useful here, see Useful addresses). If you need to use a pump it may take longer to produce the amount the baby needs. To encourage production, cut down on the amount of formula the baby is receiving, and especially the number of times the baby receives it, so that most of his feeds are from the breast.

Giving supplementary feeds in a cup or spoon can help to encourage the baby to suckle from the breast because he is not used to the teat shape and because he has not had his sucking needs met. It takes a leap of faith to do this, but remember if you did it before you can do it again. Also, if the reason you wish to relactate is because formula makes your baby ill, it is a real incentive to succeed.

BREASTFEEDING AND CONTRACEPTION

Natural Infertility while Breastfeeding

The hormones produced while breastfeeding suppress ovulation. The more often the baby feeds the more complete this effect is. So during the first six months of exclusive breastfeeding the likelihood of the mother becoming pregnant is very low. It depends on the total number of minutes nursing a day. There are of course natural variations and it probably also depends on how well the mother is fed. Our bodies are designed to successfully raise one child before going on to the next. Although it is perfectly possible to continue nursing a toddler while pregnant.

A natural period of infertility between each pregnancy gives the body a chance to recover. From the women I have met and discussed this with, the infertile period can be quite a lot longer than six months. One woman could not conceive until her eighteen month old stopped her one feed a day. After my second child I had no periods for nineteen months, and my third child did not arrive until the second was over three years old. Research has been done in conjunction with the La Leche League to discover how much a baby needs to

be nursing for the contraceptive effect to be reliable. Ovulation occurs before the first period, so you may not get obvious warning. The mucous levels change noticeably however, so you can learn to read them (look up Natural Birth Control).
Some women also find that there are very fertile as soon as they stop nursing.

This information is useful to you if, for example, you were unaware that having no periods is normal and nothing to worry about. Also you may have odd cycles, which I did, and my GP eventually said that anything is normal while breastfeeding.

The Pill

The Pill, a steroid, is known to change the whole body chemistry significantly and alter the constituents of breastmilk, so women are not generally prescribed it while breastfeeding. Some women are advised to take the mini pill, and while I would make the same observation as with the pill, I know that the hormones can interact with the body's own and result in pregnancy before the body's own period of natural infertility whilst breastfeeding has ended. It is thought that this may be a result of the two cancelling each other out. In other words women become pregnant while taking it.

The long term effect of steroid taking on a daily basis is unknown and the current concerns over infertility suggest that we need to be cautious. My opinion is that other forms of contraception that do not interfere with the milk production or affect the infant's system are preferable.

CONCLUSION

Breastfeeding is about promoting health. It is about equipping our infants to grow up in the world, preparing them directly for the culture they live in, responding to the everyday infections and bumps that they will undoubtedly experience.

It is a system designed to support the infant in every way:

1. Physically, by providing the correct nutrition for bodily development and protection from illness during infancy and by teaching the baby how to fight infection itself at any time in its life. From the lining of the gut

during the first feed when the correct gut flora is established, to identifying and destroying potential cancer cells, human milk has a very special function that should not be underestimated. Its effects last for a lifetime.

2. Emotionally, by ensuring the mother is close at hand and that the milk isn't hard for the baby to digest, making him feel miserable.

3. Mentally, by providing the best nutrients for brain and nerve development. You may be aware of the work that showed IQ levels are higher in breastfed infants. Suitable nutrition at the time of rapid brain development is bound to be important.

Also the baby is stimulated by being held, moved about and facing and being talked to by its mother.

I suspect that a dramatic increase in the breastfeeding rate would have more impact on infant health than routine antenatal care can ever have. I believe that it is more important. You cannot interfere with pregnancy as easily or dramatically as you can by giving a baby bottles of formula after the baby is born. People tend to trust the mother's body to feed her baby before it is born; why not afterwards?

Much of the knowledge our ancestors had about breastfeeding is gone and so we have to rediscover it for ourselves. It takes time to get to know our babies: each one is different. We need to allow ourselves the luxury of admitting our ignorance so that we can relax about having to get it right and allow our babies to decide how much and how often they should be fed.

The reality of breastfeeding for many women in Britain is that it is a disappointment. For whatever reason women expect labour to be long and difficult and breastfeeding to be quick and easy. It is a skill that needs to be learned and takes patience to master. Women find it confusing, time consuming and painful. While those who see the benefits and are determined to master it, do so, a greater number give up. In a society that does little to support breastfeeding women, I would like to acknowledge all those who continue because they believe that it is important to do the best for their baby. For some it is not an easy path.

The political reality of breastfeeding in this country is that the information and support structure that women need to succeed is haphazard. It needs government review, encouragement, backing and financial incentive as well as investment. Society needs to openly accept mothers breastfeeding in public. Medical carers need to be convinced of the benefits of breast milk. Realistic maternity leave (and paternity leave) needs to be developed. These are the features of the western countries where there are high rates of breastfeeding. Breastfeeding is accepted as is the notion that the mother needs to be taken care of as she nurtures her baby.

Wouldn't it be wonderful if those changes took place here too?

I hope that by reading this book you have been able to follow your instincts about nurturing your baby, in a way that you otherwise might not. I hope that you may not have been as influenced as much as you might have been by other people, who do not know as much about your baby and your priorities as you do. I hope that you have been able to enjoy your breastfeeding experience for the beautiful, warm relationship it can be.

INDEX

Useful addresses, look on website for helplines.
Association of Breastfeeding Mothers
www.abm.me.uk
La Leche League
www.laleche.org.uk
National Childbirth Trust
https://www.nct.org.uk/parenting/feeding

Catherine Holland's published books:
Rebirthing Breathwork: The making an independent adult

The Reality of Breastfeeding

That's Me! an email odyssey to find a soulmate

Indestructible Soul: How I decided not to die

eGuides
Stop Suffering Back Pain

Confidently Refuse Vaccinations

Easy Raw Main Meals

10 Keys to Unlocking Back Pain

10 Keys to Unlocking Neck Pain

10 Keys to Unlocking Hip Pain

10 Keys to Unlocking Ankle Pain

10 Keys to Unlocking Hand Pain

10 Keys to Unlocking Shoulder Pain

10 Keys to Unlocking Knee Pain

Catherine Holland is a Rebirther, trained with the Holistic Rebirthing Institute, and for many years a committee member of the British Rebirth Society. She has been teaching rebirthing breathwork for 26 years. She was a breastfeeding counsellor with the National Childbirth Trust for 19 years. She has three children. Following an accident where her leg was crushed by a car, she trained in Remedial Massage with the Northern Institute and founded a pain clinic in Oxford where she treated old injuries for 14 years until 2015. She is currently an inspiring author and virtual Breath Coach, working online with adults all over the world to be able to breathe through every experience, letting go of the past and enjoying the present. Information about her practice, articles and books can be found at www.catherineholland.co.uk

Facebook page for The Reality of Breastfeeding Book:
https://www.facebook.com/breastfeedingbook/
Feel free to ask me anything you like there.

www.ingramcontent.com/pod-product-compliance
Lightning Source LLC
Chambersburg PA
CBHW022212050726

47590CB00002B/767